Skin Cover in the Injured Hand

For Churchill Livingstone

Publisher: Simon Fathers
Project Editor: Clare Wood-Allum
Editorial Co-ordination: Editorial Resources Unit
   Copy Editor: Jennifer Bew
   Indexer: Brian Armitage
Production Controller: Neil Dickson
Design: Design Resources Unit
Sales Promotion Executive: Louise Johnstone

Skin Cover in the Injured Hand

EDITED BY

David M. Evans MB BS FRCS
Consultant Hand Surgeon,
Guy's Hospital, London and The Hand Clinic,
Oakley Green, Windsor, UK

CHURCHILL LIVINGSTONE
EDINBURGH LONDON MADRID MELBOURNE NEW YORK AND TOKYO 1992

CHURCHILL LIVINGSTONE
Medical Division of Longman Group UK Limited

Distributed in the United States of America by Churchill
Livingstone Inc., 650 Avenue of the Americas, New York,
N.Y. 10011, and by associated companies, branches and
representatives throughout the world.

First published 1992

ISBN 0-443-03799-X

British Library Cataloguing in Publication Data
A catalogue record for this book is available from the British
Library.

Library of Congress Cataloging in Publication Data
A catalog record for this book is available from the Library of
Congress.

The
publisher's
policy is to use
**paper manufactured
from sustainable forests**

Printed in Great Britain by The Bath Press, Avon

Preface

Return of hand function following injury can only be expected if all damaged structures and all gliding mechanisms are restored simultaneously. The skin is a vital component in this process, and it is fitting that a whole volume in the Hand and Upper Limb Series should be devoted to considerations of skin cover. The first, and longer, section deals with the various techniques of skin replacement currently in use. Although most established methods are included, this section is not completely comprehensive, but does attempt to give some perspective to newer techniques, such as tissue expansion and venous flaps, to provide detailed descriptions of important basic techniques – free grafts, local flaps and free flaps – and to evaluate the current place of less used procedures such as distant pedicle flaps.

In the second section, the hand is divided into areas which have distinct requirements in terms of skin cover, and the various techniques are evaluated in that context. In this way, it is hoped that the trainee and the practising surgeon can rapidly find reference to a particular clinical problem, and at the same time find descriptions of the techniques selected.

Every injured hand demands some attention to the specialized skin envelope which maintains its internal environment. The three vital requirements for skin function are blood supply, sensation and mobility in all directions. Techniques are continuously evolving to satisfy these, and it is hoped that this book will provide a useful current view of this important area of hand surgery. Sincere gratitude is due to the authors, who have enthusiastically contributed.

Windsor   D.M.E.
1992

Contributors

Marc Bissonnette MD
Formerly Christine Kleinert Fellow in Hand Surgery, University of Louisville School of Medicine, Louisville, Kentucky, USA; Currently Hand Surgeon, Montreal, Quebec, Canada

Michael J. M. Black MB BS FRCS
Consultant Plastic and Reconstructive Surgeon, The Royal Victoria Infirmary, Newcastle upon Tyne, UK

Warren Breidenbach MD
Assistant Clinical Professor of Surgery (Plastic and Reconstructive), University of Louisville School of Medicine, Louisville, Kentucky, USA

Dieter Buck-Gramcko MD FRCPS
Chief, Department of Hand and Plastic Surgery, Berufsgenossenschaftliches Unfallkrankenhaus, Hamburg; Associate Professor of Hand and Plastic Surgery, University of Hamburg Medical School, Hamburg, Germany

N. Citron MD
Former Resident, Emergency Hand Unit (SOS Main), Strasbourg, France

John Colville FRCS(Edin) FRCSI
Consultant Plastic and Hand Surgeon, Royal Victoria and Ulster Hospitals, Belfast, UK

David M. Evans MB BS FRCS
Consultant Hand Surgeon, Guy's Hospital, London and The Hand Clinic, Oakley Green, Windsor, UK

Guy Foucher MD
Ancien Chef de Clinique, Head of the Emergency Hand Unit (SOS Main), Strasbourg, France

David Gault MB ChB FRCS
Consultant Plastic Surgeon, Mount Vernon Hospital, Northwood, Middlesex, UK

Alan M. Godfrey MA FRCS(Edin)
Consultant Plastic and Reconstructive Surgeon, Oxford; Honorary Consultant Plastic Surgeon to Oxford and Swindon Hospitals, Oxford and Swindon, UK

Anders Hedlund MD
Burns Unit, Department of Plastic and Hand Surgery, Uppsala University Hospital, Uppsala, Sweden

Sune Johansson MD
Associate Professor, Department of Plastic and Hand Surgery, Uppsala University Hospital, Uppsala, Sweden

James Katsaros MB BS FRACS
Senior Visiting Plastic Surgeon, Royal Adelaide Hospital; Honorary Plastic Surgeon, Adelaide Children's Hospital, Adelaide, South Australia

Christopher Khoo FRCS
Consultant Plastic Surgeon, Wexham Park and Heatherwood NHS Trust, East Berkshire, UK

Derek Mercer FRCS(T)
Consultant Plastic Surgeon, King's College Hospital, London, UK

Arthur MacG. Morris MA MB FRCS(Edin) FRCS(Eng)
Consultant Plastic Surgeon, Tayside Health Board; Honorary Senior Lecturer, The Medical School, Dundee University, Dundee, UK

Paul J. Smith FRCS
Consultant Plastic and Hand Surgeon, Mount Vernon Hospital, Northwood, Middlesex and Hospitals for Sick Children, Great Ormond Street, London, UK

Tsu-Min Tsai MD
Associate Clinical Professor of Surgery, University of Louisville School of Medicine, Louisville, Kentucky, USA

Joseph Upton MD
Clinical Associate Professor of Surgery, Harvard Medical School, Boston, Massachusetts, USA

John Walton FRACS
Commonwealth Senior Registrar, Department of Plastic Surgery, Mount Vernon Hospital, Northwood, Middlesex, UK

Joanne Werntz MD
Formerly Hand Scholar, Christine Kleinert Institute of Hand and Microsurgery, University of Louisville School of Medicine, Louisville, Kentucky; Currently Director of Hand Surgery, Orlando Regional Medical Center, Orlando, Florida, USA

Contents

M. J. M. Black

Wound care and skin closure

Primary wound healing is always the paramount goal in the management of the injured hand. Delayed healing predisposes to oedema, sepsis, excess scarring and joint stiffness (Beasley 1981). Every wound, even if unsuitable for actual primary closure, must be prepared for closure at the earliest possible opportunity.

WOUND TYPES

Rank, Wakefield and Hueston (1973) made the distinction between 'tidy' and 'untidy' wounds, as a classification to guide the surgeon in the management of a particular wound (Rank et al 1973). The crucial factor is the state of viability of the tissues surrounding the wound. This is, of course, related principally to the mechanism of injury, for example incision, crush, avulsion or burning. Only the first of these would seem to result in wounds suitable for immediate primary closure, without risking the onset of sepsis, and with any hope of actual primary

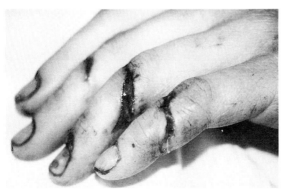

Fig. 1.1 Clean lacerations.

healing (Fig. 1.1). Most wounds, however, may, by suitable intervention, be converted into a state at least suitable for delayed, if not actual, primary closure. Such intervention may result in a wound that can only be closed by some means of tissue transfer. If this leads to primary healing, it is vastly preferable to secondary healing following sepsis and the breakdown of the inappropriate direct suture of an unsuitable wound.

WOUND EVALUATION AND PREPARATION

The history of the injury thus indicates to a large extent the nature of the problem, but the course of action is always the same: to prepare the wound for successful closure at the earliest possible moment. Many wounds involve deep structures as well as skin, and primary repair of these is also most desirable. In this situation uncomplicated wound healing is doubly important, if the deep repairs are not to be compromised.

Adequate wound inspection and preparation require anaesthesia and control of haemorrhage. Nerve block anaesthesia is often suitable. For digital wounds a distal block may be adequate, but the need to tolerate the application of a proximal tourniquet indicates the use of brachial plexus block in many cases. Intravenous regional anaesthesia is largely unsuitable, as the effect is lost as soon as the tourniquet is released. General anaesthesia is a very acceptable alternative, largely essential for children, and perhaps also when the need for tissue transfer from distant sites is anticipated.

The tourniquet is of exceptional value in all hand

surgery: it is not often that the added period of tissue ischaemia resulting from its use is of any real significance. The proximal pneumatic type will be the one used most, because of its safety and reliability. Digital tourniquets should be of the flat, broad elastic type, to avoid local damage. It is wise to release the tourniquet to allow haemostasis, prior to wound closure: this is because haematoma is a potent cause of later problems, including pain, sepsis and added fibrosis. Reinflation of the tourniquet for the actual closure can be helpful as it eliminates the oozing associated with suturing and the dependent position required at that stage.

Once anaesthesia has been achieved and haemorrhage controlled, wound cleansing is begun. This process is undertaken by the surgeon personally, as it provides a great opportunity to assess the wound at the same time. The whole hand is carefully washed before the wound itself receives attention – it is probably wise to use a physiological saline solution containing a mild antiseptic. The skin is cleaned with soap and, if necessary, a scrubbing brush. The limb is then formally prepared and draped. The wound is copiously irrigated with saline to remove contaminants in the form of dirt, foreign materials, blood clots and loose devitalized tissue, and careful exploration is undertaken to ensure that no such material is missed. A thorough assessment is made of the tissues around the wound and their vitality. Obviously dead and grossly contaminated tissue is removed. Under most circumstances the hand, like the face, has an excellent blood supply, so that formal excision of all wound edges is not required. Release of the tourniquet may be necessary to evaluate the state of tissue perfusion before deciding upon the extent of any excision required.

Many wounds will have to be extended to provide access to deep structures. The guidelines governing the planning of incisions into the hand are as follows:

1. Adequate exposure must be achieved
2. The blood supply of the tissues must be preserved
3. The incision must not predispose to later contracture, i.e. it must, if at all possible, follow lines that do not change length, during flexion and extension.

The latter is particularly important on the flexor surface as these scars will be relaxed for the majority of the time, whereas extensor scars tend to be kept under some tension even during rest. To gain access to the flexor surface of the fingers any combination of zigzag and mid-lateral incisions may be used (Figs 1.2, 1.3, 1.4), incorporating the traumatic wound (Fig. 1.5). The planning is often made unusually difficult because the first, traumatic, incisions were made in the wrong place!

The term 'mid-lateral' is generally accepted, but is in fact inaccurate. The intention is that the incision should join the axes of motion of the joints: as the skeleton lies quite dorsally in the digits, this line will not actually be mid-lateral. In practice it has been shown to be unnecessary to take the tips of zigzag flaps as far as the lateral line, thus reducing the risk of tip necrosis. The integrity of the digital artery at the base of such flaps is important and

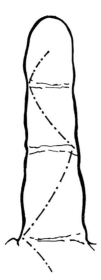

Fig. 1.2 Volar zigzag incision.

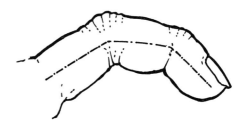

Fig. 1.3 Lateral incision.

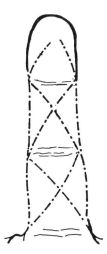

Fig. 1.4 Composite diagram of the various possible volar and lateral incisions. Suitable combinations may be used.

should be considered during planning. In the palm a combination of stepped longitudinal and transverse incisions is suitable (Fig. 1.6). It should be remembered that the blood supply of the palmar skin is such that extensive flaps must be raised with great caution. On the dorsal surface the flap length should be restricted and the incisions more straight than zigzag (Fig. 1.7), to preserve the blood supply and because contracture is less of a problem. Transverse lacerations at the wrist with deep structures divided require longitudinal

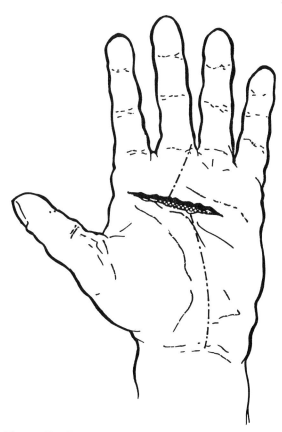

Fig. 1.6 Possible extension of a palmar wound. This may be connected to zigzag incisions in any finger.

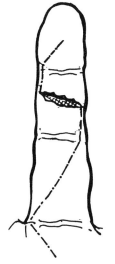

Fig. 1.5 An example of extension of a volar wound.

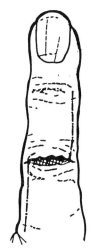

Fig. 1.7 Extension of a dorsal wound.

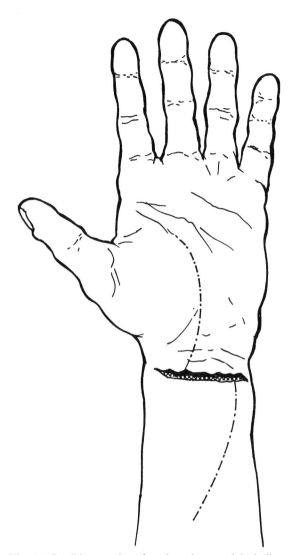

Fig. 1.8 Possible extension of a volar wrist wound, including division of the volar carpal ligament.

another. It is important to realize that in certain circumstances, however, it might not be suitable to proceed to wound closure. These are the situations where the tissue vitality cannot be accurately assessed, or may actually be expected to decline with the passage of time. The classic situation of this type is the blast or high-velocity missile wound, where progressive tissue necrosis may almost be expected. More commonly, this situation is seen where the injuring agent has caused crush, avulsion or burning, or even a combination of these, as in the 'hot moulding press' injury.

It is vital not to lose sight of the stated aim of achieving early wound healing under these circumstances. It is correct, however, not to close the wound but to protect the exposed tissues from desiccation and contamination by an appropriate dressing, until it is possible to be sure that all devitalized tissue has been excised. What this means in practical terms is that the wound has to be reinspected under anaesthesia in, say, 48 hours' time. If doubt still remains, the procedure is repeated a further 48 hours later, the wound being closed as part of that procedure if at all possible.

Haemostasis is achieved by the ligation of large vessels and the use of bipolar coagulation of the smaller bleeding points. Unipolar diathermy is too destructive to be ideal in hand surgery, the heating effect of the current being propagated quite widely into the surrounding tissues.

WOUND CLOSURE

If possible direct wound closure is undertaken, but this must not further compromise the tissue perfusion. What this implies is that excessive tension across the wound is unacceptable. It must also be remembered that a degree of oedema is inevitable in the early stages of wound healing, and this will add to the original tension. The author found that the common wrist and forearm wounds can usually be successfully closed directly after repair of the deep structures.

If tensionless direct closure cannot be achieved, then a skin graft or flap is indicated. A free skin graft will only 'take' on a viable recipient bed – this is sometimes described as a bed that if left, would produce granulation tissue. Such suitable beds

exposure. The incisions may be gently curving in each direction, and do not necessarily need to begin at each lateral extent of the original wound – the flaps may otherwise be excessively long for the available blood supply. If near the wrist, a formal decompression of the carpal tunnel will become part of the exposure, and is indicated to cope with the swelling associated with tendon and nerve healing (Fig. 1.8).

Once cleansing, excision, deep repair and haemostasis have been achieved the wound will be suitable for primary closure by one means or comprise, for example, muscle, paratenon and periosteum, but even anastomosed vessels are sufficiently vital to ensure the 'take' of a free skin graft. Such grafts may not be sufficiently thick or durable to be the permanent repair, but often such a simple technique will achieve the object in mind: early wound healing.

Where the wound will not provide conditions suitable for a skin graft, a flap, with its independent blood supply, will be essential. Sometimes, as implied above, flap repair will be more suitable than a free graft from the point of view of long-term function, rather than because it is essential for wound healing. Another indication for flap cover is where later surgery on the underlying structures is anticipated, for example, nerve grafting. This is to provide a nutritious bed for the free nerve grafts, and because previously placed skin grafts cannot be lifted for access and returned in the way that a flap can.

Very many types of dressing have been advocated for the temporary cover of exposed tissues, including biological dressings. The requirements are a dressing that will protect the wound from further contamination, prevent desiccation and preferably be non-adherent. The best in the biological field is fresh autogenous split-thickness skin graft, the use of which is sometimes justified even if it is to be discarded later. The potential value of lyophilized xenograft seems to be countered by its considerable expense. Most often a simple dressing, such as vaseline gauze and saline-moistened gauze is perfectly adequate.

Suturing

The purpose of suturing is to draw the skin edges into apposition and to maintain this situation until healing is sufficiently advanced for the sutures to be removed. It is important to realize that skin apposition implies more than just epidermal apposition. If only that is achieved, then primary healing may not occur, because the broader skin interfaces are not in contact and because the dead space beneath the epidermis will fill with blood or exudate, which will probably result in sepsis. The various classic suture styles are designed to prevent such problems.

In the hand, deep subcutaneous sutures are

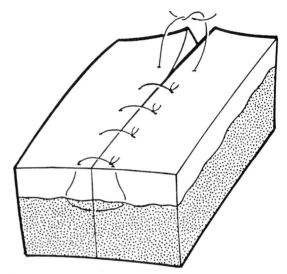

Fig. 1.9 Simple interrupted sutures.

hardly ever required, but if they are needed, they should preferably be absorbable, and their knots placed deeply. Black silk is the traditional suture material for the skin, but it displays sufficient disadvantages when compared with modern monofilament materials as to be relatively undesirable. Monofilament nylon is an excellent material which is very inert and does not exhibit capillarity to the same damaging extent. The most frequently suitable suture sizes are 4/0 and 5/0. The use of

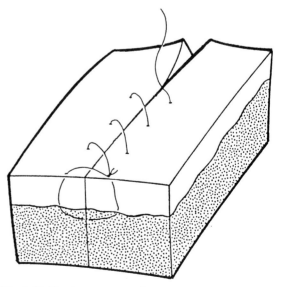

Fig. 1.10 Continuous over-and-over suture.

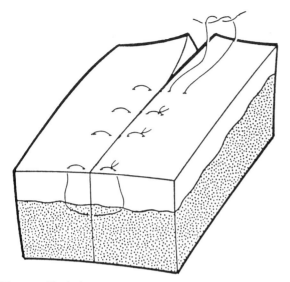

Fig. 1.11 Vertical mattress sutures.

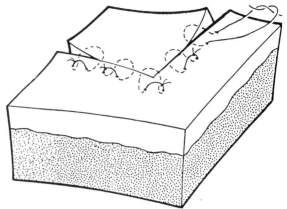

Fig. 1.12 Half-buried horizontal mattress sutures.

absorbable material as a skin suture is acceptable in children, but less so in adults as it may linger and leave suture tracks.

Most of the various suture styles have their place in hand surgery. The simple interrupted suture (Fig. 1.9) is usually suitable, especially on the palmar surface and digits. Continuous over-and-over sutures (Fig. 1.10) are similarly applicable, especially where the wound is straight and long. The skin of the dorsum of the hand and of the forearm has a tendency to invert: this can be prevented by the use of vertical mattress sutures (Fig. 1.11), but these may leave conspicuous marks if they are too tight or are left in too long. Half-buried horizontal mattress sutures (Fig. 1.12) have a special place where wounds are ragged, or where the corners of flaps are to be inset, because the buried half has a relatively sparing effect upon the blood supply of the tissues, in addition to the suture's mechanical advantages at corners. Continuous subcuticular sutures (Fig. 1.13) leave no marks, prevent inversion and may be left in longer for wound support if desired. If they are made of absorbable material they need not be removed at all. Of the non-absorbable sutures, Prolene (Ethicon) pulls out more easily than nylon. Even though Dexon (Davies & Geck) and Vicryl (polyglactin 910–Ethicon) have been criticized for causing reactions in this situation, it is the author's experience that so long as knots near

the surface are avoided, this is not really a problem. However a better material by far is PDS (polydioxanone–Ethicon), in view of its extreme inertness and solubility. Adhesive skin strips are useful in conjunction with subcuticular sutures, and indeed on their own, as long as one remembers that they tend to draw only the epidermal edges together, rather than the depth of the wound interface.

Drains are not often required, but if dead space exists with the risk of haematoma formation, a suction drain would be preferable. Simple, soft

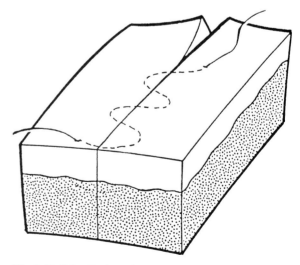

Fig. 1.13 Subcuticular suture.

rubber drains are useful where dead space tends to be closed by natural tissue tension.

DRESSINGS

The purpose of a dressing is to protect, to splint and to absorb exudate or discharge. Against the wound itself should be a non-adherent porous layer; next should be an absorbent material. The method of splintage is open to much variation, depending upon the extent and type of the injury, and upon individual preferences. Circumferential bandages can be used to good effect over suitable padding, but great care has to be taken to avoid excessive compression, especially proximally, where the tourniquet effect would contribute to oedema. Plaster of Paris slabs, either palmar or dorsal, are easy to apply and are secure, but the same comments apply to the bandages required to hold them in place. The potentially least constricting of all is a circumferential plaster cast, but this should be split if there is any possibility of swelling.

POST-OPERATIVE CARE

Perhaps the most immediate postoperative danger is the formation of oedema. If excessive and prolonged, this can have a most damaging effect upon the hand, leading to fibrosis, joint stiffness and tendon adhesions. Prevention is best, but if oedema does occur, it must be reduced as a priority. Elevation is the principal means in the early stages, but movement is in fact the most essential and natural mechanism. The injured hand should be immobilized for the shortest possible time, and those parts that do not need to be immobilized should not be immobilized. The position chosen for immobilization is of considerable importance in the prevention of complications. The ideal position of the joints has often to be modified when the protection of deep repairs is overriding. The metacarpophalangeal joints are best immobilized in flexion, as in that position the collateral ligaments are taut and therefore cannot become contracted. The interphalangeal joints are safest in the extended position as the accessory collateral ligaments will then be taut. Wrist extension tends

to place all these joints into their ideal positions through the tenodesis effect on the long tendons, and is thus the key to correct positioning. If movement of a particular joint does not stress or excessively disturb a wound, then it need not, and should not, be immobilized unless deep repairs require otherwise. Some wounds in lines of election, as outlined above, may not require immobilization at all, and this is certainly acceptable when the mobilization of other structures is a priority. For skin wounds alone, whatever splintage is used may be discarded after suture removal at the latest. Persistent oedema can be dissipated by a skilled physiotherapist, assisted, if necessary, by the use of pneumatic compression devices.

Elevation can be achieved by means varying from drip stands to slings. The common triangular sling is, unfortunately, often far from elevating! High elevation lowers the arterial input pressure, so a compromise sometimes has to be found, as, for example, where the patency of microvascular anastomoses is a competing priority.

Dressings may be left in place until suture removal is due provided they are not soaked through with blood or exudate or until it is appropriate to allow less restricted movement. Suture removal may be undertaken at 10 days or so, but if disturbance at that stage is undesirable, the removal of such inert materials as those recommended may safely be deferred.

ANTIBIOTICS

The use of prophylactic antibiotics is somewhat controversial. In the case of clean-cut wounds with no significant devitalization of the tissues, there is little risk of sepsis developing so long as wound management has followed the advice given above. The author does not, however, believe that the practice could be criticized in any individual case and the requirements of tetanus prophylaxis must not be forgotten.

However, when the vitality of the tissues is impaired, or contamination has been severe, the prescription of antibiotics is appropriate. An anti-staphylococcal penicillin combined with an anti-anaerobe (e.g.metronidazole) would seem to be reasonable.

SPECIAL WOUNDS

Certain wound types require extra comment, although careful application of the principles already outlined will be indicated.

Burst lacerations

These are caused by forceful impact. The tissues are ruptured in a ragged fashion and there may be devitalization of surrounding skin (Figs 1.14, 1.15). Careful but conservative excision is required, and probably not primary closure. If sutures are inserted they must not create undue tension. Adhesive strips are sometime acceptable in this situation. A skin graft should be applied if the wound is of significant size.

Crush injuries

These are often very severe, as there is extensive tissue damage, the extent of which is difficult to assess initially (Fig. 1.15). Primary closure is therefore rarely advisable, and efforts are directed to decompression rather than suture, although skin grafts may be applied quite early. High elevation to control oedema is important. The dependent position required for distant flap application is a disadvantage. A microvascular free flap may be a better choice.

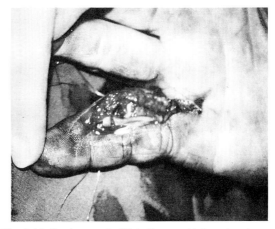

Fig. 1.15 Crush wound of little finger, with bursting element.

Avulsion and degloving injuries (Figs 1.16, 1.17, 1.18)

Although both mechanisms may be involved, the separation of large flaps from their blood supply is of greater significance than crushing. Large areas of specialized skin are involved, and the vascular compromise of the flaps is potentially progressive. Caution is therefore required. Theoretically it might be possible to restore the blood supply by microvascular anastomosis, perhaps using vein grafts: 'ring avulsion' is a practical example where this approach has proved successful. Otherwise successive excisions and appropriate skin replace-

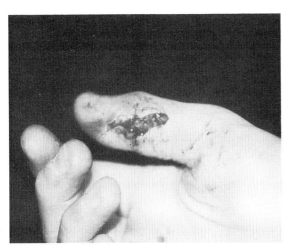

Fig. 1.14 Burst wound of thumb.

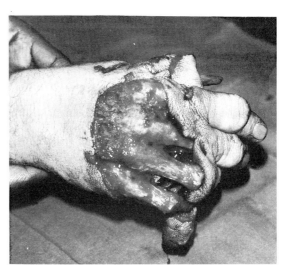

Fig. 1.16 Avulsion of skin of fingers.

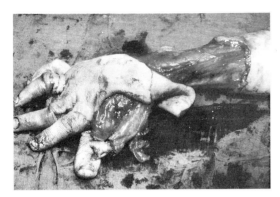

Fig. 1.17 Major crush/avulsion injury.

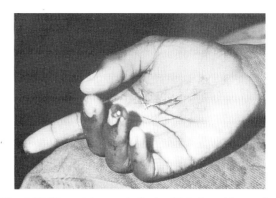

Fig. 1.19 Clean stab wound of palm. Note the evidence of tendon severance.

ment are required. Distally based palmar flaps are an especially serious problem, because the skin is so specialized and the anatomy of the blood supply so unfavourable.

Puncture wounds

It is often difficult to decide how seriously to treat small puncture wounds. Obviously if damage to the deep structures is recognized, exploration will be required (Fig. 1.l9). If there seems to be risk that dirt has been impregnated then a similar approach is necessary. Primary closure of the extended wound will follow if conditions are suitable.

Friction injuries

The problems here are similar to burn injuries, with the addition of impregnation of dirt (Fig. 1.20). It is most important to remove this to avoid tattooing,

which is very difficult or impossible to remove once the wound has healed. This is achieved by scrubbing. Otherwise the wound is treated similarly to a mixed-depth burn excision, with replacement of devitalized skin as soon as this can be recognized.

Multiple parallel lacerations

These are often self-inflicted. The problem is the possibility of necrosis of intervening skin, which may be worsened by attempts to suture such wounds. If the skin is alive, closure may be achieved by a combination of subcuticular suturing and the simple application of skin tapes and dressings.

Bites

These are injuries for which antibiotic therapy is indicated. *Staphylococcus aureus* is the most

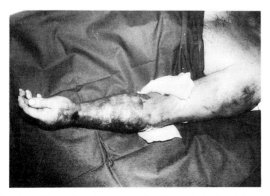

Fig. 1.18 Extensive closed crush/avulsion/degloving injury caused by a conveyer belt. All of the forearm skin necrosed.

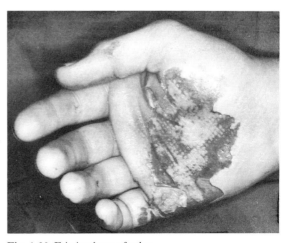

Fig. 1.20 Friction burn of palm.

common infecting organism, so flucloxacillin is probably the best choice.

Animal bites are less potentially serious than human bites. If treated early primary closure is usually permissible.

Human bites have a far more sinister reputation, and should be treated by debridement and delayed closure. Often the bite is more correctly called 'fist on teeth' injury: this is the situation where compound injuries of the metacarpo-phalangeal joints occur, sometimes with fragments of broken teeth left in the joint. Recognition of this problem is the first step in proper management, followed by adequate surgical exploration.

REFERENCES

Beasley R W 1981 Hand injuries. Saunders, Philadelphia
Rank B K, Wakefield A R, Hueston J T 1973 Surgery of repair as applied to hand injuries, 4th edn. Williams & Wilkins, Baltimore

C. T. K. Khoo (with illustrations by D. T. Gault, FRCS)

2 Free skin grafts

HISTORY

The first documented description of completely successful skin grafting to the hand was given by Sir Astley Cooper in 1827:

'I amputated a thumb for a patient in Guy's Hospital, and finding that I had not preserved a sufficient quantity of skin to cover the stump, I cut out a piece from the thumb which I had removed, and applied it upon the stump, confining it by stripes of adhesive plaister. On taking off the dressings a few days after the operation I found that the portion which had been completely separated, and afterwards placed upon the stump, was firmly united and organized.'

Other surgeons were apparently unaware of this case, and skin grafting was not reestablished as a surgical technique for some 50 years.

In 1863, Bert described the use of experimental skin grafts in his medical thesis, and suggested that the technique could be used in humans. Reverdin's initial attempts at skin grafting (Reverdin 1869) used very thin skin in small fragments – 'greffes épidermiques'. In 1874, Magnier described the use of these epidermic grafts to resurface a large avulsion injury of the back of the hand (Magnier 1874). Thin razor-cut grafts and the introduction of skin grafting are usually credited to Thiersch, although he did not publish his description until 1886. Ollier emphasized the importance of the dermis, and was successful in transferring thicker grafts containing dermis

('greffes cutanées') which were of a useful size, up to 8 cm² and provided a better quality of skin cover (Ollier 1872). He went on to graft full-thickness skin as though the technique did not become common until Wolfe's description in 1875.

STRUCTURE AND FUNCTION: THE SKIN OF THE HAND

The skin of the hand is specially adapted to its functional role, being delicately sensate yet capable of secure and powerful grasp. There are basic differences between the skin on the palmar and dorsal aspects of the hand, and also a unique specialization of the fingertips in the pulps and nails.

The volar skin is thicker than the dorsal skin (Fig. 2.1). It is relatively non-elastic and is stabilized through its attachments to the underlying skeleton, to prevent slipping and shearing whilst

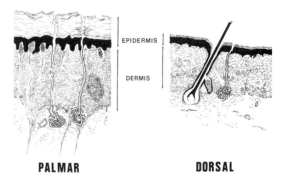

Fig. 2.1 The different thicknesses of palmar and dorsal skin are illustrated in this comparative diagram, where histological sections from the same subject have been drawn to the same scale.

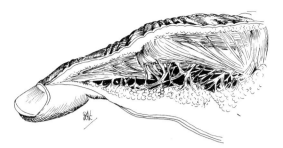

Fig. 2.2 The palmar (volar) skin is stabilized through extensive fibrous attachments through the fibrous septa, and the ligaments of Cleland. (Drawn from a dissection.)

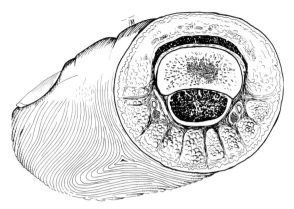

Fig. 2.3 Cross-section through the terminal phalanx of a finger, illustrating the fibrous septa. (Drawn from a dissection.)

grasping. Movement on the volar aspect is absorbed in the flexion creases. Deep fixation is achieved in the fingers through the fibrous septa and ligaments of Cleland, and through the attachments of the palmar skin to the palmar fascia and thence to the deep intermetacarpal ligaments (Fig. 2.2). This anatomical pattern of skin attachment is reflected in the pattern of skin avulsion following shearing injury or degloving. On the palm a thick layer of skin and fascia is raised at a subfascial level where the attachment to the synovial layer is weakest (McGregor 1970), while on the dorsum of the hand the lax and mobile skin is ripped off at a subdermal plane, often suffering extensive necrosis following vascular damage.

The volar skin is hairless, whereas the dorsal skin supports hair as far as the distal interphalangeal joints in 90% of people, and the hair always grows obliquely and points to the ulnar side (Barron 1970). The quality and characteristics of skin on the hand are affected by the patient's occupation.

The finger pulps are highly specialized in structure (Fig. 2.3). The skin is bound down by deeply running connective tissue septa which lobulate and stabilize the subcutaneous adipose tissue, so that the skin does not slide or slip over the terminal phalanx. The pulp skin is marked by a pattern of dermatoglyphs, or papillary ridges, richly supplied with the openings of sweat glands which moisten the pulp skin to increase tactile adhesion.

Although the melanocyte density varies between the palmar (1680 ± 440) and dorsal (2200 ± 600) surfaces of the hand (Fitzpatrick & Szabo 1959) the pigmentation difference is mainly due to differences in melanocyte activity. The use of the plantar donor site has been found to be cosmetically very satisfactory for resurfacing the palm in patients with pigmented skin.

The palmar surface of the hand is richly supplied with nerve endings. Meissner's corpuscles are tactile end-organs located in the dermal papillae, and their distribution (and therefore the sensitivity of the skin) varies along the length of the digits (Wood-Jones 1942) (Table 2.1).

Vater–Pacini corpuscles are large pressure receptors situated in the deep dermis or the superficial part of the subcutis. They measure up to 1 mm in diameter and are found in the palm, often adjacent to nerves. Of the 2000 Pacinian corpuscles present in the body, some 800 are present in the fingers (Barron 1970).

It is a basic principle in reconstructive hand surgery that lost skin should be replaced with tissue that is as like the original as possible. On the palmar surface of the hand, for example, (and when a satisfactory vascular bed is preserved) a skin graft replacement from a like area of skin such as the sole, offers a better approximation to the normal anatomy of the palm than resurfacing with a thick pedicled flap, which may only provide a

Table 2.1 Distribution of Meissner's corpuscles (Wood-Jones, 1942)

Meissner's corpuscles per mm²	
Distal pulp	50/mm²
Middle phalanx	20/mm²
Proximal phalanx	10/mm²

Table 2.2 Histological structure of palmar and dorsal skin (Ward & Ecclestone, 1985)

Histological structure	Plantar or palmar skin	Dorsal hand or foot skin
S. corneum	thick layer to stand pressure	medium thickness flexible
S. granulosum	thick layer of keratohyaline granules	thinner layer keratohyaline granules
Rete ridges	numerous, deep dermal papillae	shallow ridges with papillae
Melanocytes	dense & inactive (little pigment)	very dense (basal layer pigmented)
Elastic fibres	numerous	sparse
Pilosebaceous units	none	present
Sweat glands	abundant	sparse
Vascularity	poor	rich
Colour	pale	darker

slippery skin surface, and which is less well adapted to grasp. The skin on the palm of the hand is very similar to the skin of the sole of the foot. The histological differences between palmar and dorsal hand skin are similar to the differences between plantar and dorsal foot skin and have been summarized in Table 2.2 (Ward & Ecclestone 1985).

MECHANISMS OF SKIN-GRAFT TAKE

The clinical stages in the healing of a skin graft are now well recognized, and were clearly described in Medawar's classic studies (Medawar 1944, 1945). Immediately after grafting the skin is pale and white, but successful take is then indicated by the development of a pink colour in the graft, with blanching and refilling on pressure. Within the first few days the epithelium may double in thickness; by the 3rd day intense mitotic activity is visible on histological sections. Epithelial cell proliferation continues, with a progressive increase in epidermal thickness of up to seven times that of the original. Surface crusting on a graft reflects the desquamation resulting from the intense mitotic activity which generates many layers of cells.

In full-thickness skin grafts there may be surface blistering and loss of epithelium as a consequence of inadequate blood supply (Hinshaw & Miller 1965), and it is well accepted that the thicker the graft, the less likely it is to achieve a complete and

uniform take (Byars 1942). The histological stages in graft healing have been exhaustively reviewed by Rudolph & Klein (1973) and Šmahel (1977). When a skin graft is placed on a vascular bed the initial phase of plasmatic imbibition is a period of varying duration during which tissue fluid and contained nutrients are absorbed, and the skin graft may gain 40% in weight. It is believed that initial revascularization occurs by inosculation: the chance matching of vascular lumina with immediate restoration of flow, and later by capillary ingrowth into the graft (Fig. 2.4).

These traditional views are supported by current experience. Clinically, it has been shown that full-thickness skin-graft take can be enhanced if attempts are made to preserve the preexisting subcutaneous vasculature, so that when the graft is placed into the recipient site the vessels in the bed are able to link up with the graft vessels to provide immediate conduits for vascular perfusion (Tsukuda 1980). Using the preserved skin vascular network (PSVN) technique, blood appeared in the graft vessels at 24 hours, and resumed circulation in the graft vessels with vascular distension has been confirmed 3 days after transplantation. These observations have been elegantly confirmed by scanning electron microscopy studies (Okada 1986) of corrosion casts, which show vascular connections developing between the graft and its bed at 3 days, with well-developed revascularization clearly established at 5 days.

A knowledge of the stages of revascularization is essential to the management of hand injuries. The initial management of a skin graft requires firm

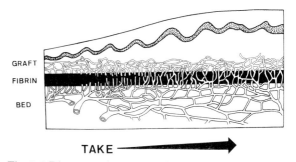

Fig. 2.4 Diagrammatic representation of the progression of skin-graft take, illustrating the thickening of the graft, with progressive capillary ingrowth through the fibrin layer between the graft and its bed.

planar contact between the graft and its bed, but prolonged splintage of the hand and wrist will lead to stiffness and swelling. It is therefore reassuring that under ideal conditions circulation begins to be established in a skin graft 3 days after transplantation from the donor site. Grafts on the hand may therefore be inspected early, at 3 or 4 days, and if the clinical appearances are satisfactory gentle mobilization may begin. Movement should be avoided before this time because the delicate neovasculature is susceptible to rupture from shearing forces. A convenient technical device to allow removal for inspection and reapplication of a bolus pressure dressing over a skin graft is the Burd button (Burd 1984) which allows the tie-over suture ends to be gathered together, released and retightened over the dressing when the skin graft has been inspected. An alternative technique is to suture a sheet of polyurethane foam over the tulle gras covering the skin graft: this provides sustained pressure on the graft and movement may be commenced with the dressing in place at 4 days. Šmahel (1965) has demonstrated that newly formed vascular anastomoses between the bed and the graft may rupture, causing a late haematoma which may result in the loss of a graft which had already begun to take. This complication may be avoided by adequate compression of the graft on to its base, or by the use of fibrin adhesive.

REINNERVATION OF GRAFTED SKIN

When grafting skin as a permanent replacement for lost tissue it is important to try to match as closely as possible the characteristics of the original skin in terms of thickness, subcutaneous padding and the presence of adnexal and sensory organs.

The recovery of sensation in grafted skin has been the subject of careful study. Following a successful take, touch, pain temperature and two-point discrimination return at different rates (Ponten 1960). Touch and two-point discrimination were found to be the most reliable indicators of the extent of reinnervation, and in all types of skin grafts the sensory pattern achieved in the graft closely matches that of the recipient site.

Full-thickness skin grafts achieve better sensation than split-thickness grafts, though recovery is slower.

Reinnervation proceeds as nerve ends in the recipient site grow in from the base and margins of the graft and migrate towards the centre, either along empty neurilemmal sheaths (Fitzgerald et al 1967) or in response to chemotactic attraction from target organs (Waris et al 1983). Specific histochemical studies suggest that ingrowing nerve ends may not reach and reconnect with the original end-organs, and that the apices of regenerating nerves may themselves function as sensory receptors (Waris 1978). The return of sweating in a graft has long been known to correlate with the return of sensation (Conway 1939), and Waris et al (1983) have now demonstrated the specific reinnervation of eccrine sweat glands, hair follicles and erector pili muscles, provided these structures are present in the grafted skin. It is therefore particularly important when selecting donor sites for skin to be grafted on the hand to provide graft tissue that is best able to substitute for the missing area of skin.

Cold sensitivity is the first thermal sensation to appear in a skin graft (Waris et al 1989). Sensation to warm and hot stimuli returns later, though not in every case. When warm sensation is recovered, threshold values for sensitivity approach normal discrimination. However, the recovery of sensation takes several years, and patients examined 2–3 years after grafting had steadily improving sensation which had not achieved normal sensitivity. The patient with skin grafts on the hand should therefore be made aware of the very significant lack of thermal sensitivity during the period of healing, and should make conscious efforts to protect against the possibility of injury in the insensate area.

SKIN GRAFT CONTRACTION: MESHED GRAFTS

The dermis is elastic, and when a skin graft is removed from its donor site it shrinks in area. This 'primary contraction' is greatest for full-thickness skin (44% of original area), intermediate for medium-thickness skin (22%) and least for very thin grafts (<10%), while true epidermal grafts do not undergo primary shrinkage (Davis & Kitlowski 1931). Full-thickness or Wolfe grafts should therefore be cut to a precise pattern, so that they may be stretched out to their normal size and tension when transferred to the recipient site.

At a later stage, following a succesful 'take' a different form of shrinkage occurs within the margins of the wound. This 'secondary contraction' is greatest in thin grafts, which will contract unless firmly adherent to an unyielding bed such as periosteum. Full-thickness skin grafts contract minimally and may be specially selected for this reason. After a slight initial contraction, full-thickness skin expands and grows with the recipient site, so that it can exceed its original size. (Ragnell 1953), and this makes full-thickness skin most suitable for use in children.

Meshed split-thickness grafts may be cut with a roller blade (Tanner et al 1964), or in a flat-bed meshing machine such as the Zimmer Meshgraft II, when the sheet of skin graft is supported on a ribbed board (Fig. 2.5). Care must be taken when using meshgraft boards to ensure that the skin is placed with the ribbed surface facing upwards against the blades: otherwise the blades will finely shred the skin into parallel strips of 'spaghetti'. Browne (1988) has, however, suggested that 'spaghetti mesh' is the most suitable form of graft for flexion creases. Grafts meshed by hand will also expand if the cuts are correctly positioned. Stretched out (expanded) meshed grafts contract more than split-thickness graft applied as a sheet. In an experimental study (Petry & Wortham 1986), wounds covered with meshed grafts originally two-thirds the area of the defect and expanded to fit (mesh ratio 1:1.5), contracted to 55% of their original size, whilst wounds covered by non-meshed grafts contracted to 81.5%.

Meshed grafts may be chosen for treatment of skin loss on the hands (for example, when burns of the hands are part of a generalized burn injury and there is a general shortage of skin), but it must then be anticipated that significant graft contracture may occur. More often, meshed grafts are used in order that graft take might be enhanced by the drainage of exudate through the skin meshes, to prevent a fluid collection under a graft which would lift it from contact with its bed. Skin expanded more than 1.5:1 is likely to produce an unfavourable cosmetic result, and adequate drainage is achieved if the graft is meshed and placed in the defect without expansion. Smaller pieces of

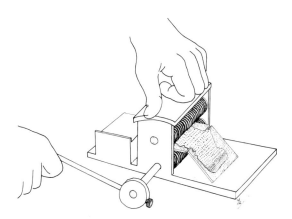

Fig. 2.5 A flat-bed skin-graft meshing machine. The skin is placed on a diagonally-ribbed plastic carrier board, and passed through parallel roller blades which produce an even pattern of staggered cuts allowing expansion of the skin when tension is applied at right-angles to the line of the cut. The skin may be placed against the carrier board epidermis down or epidermis up, according to preference. However, if the skin is placed epidermis side down, against the board, it may be taken directly from the mesher and directly applied to the raw area still lying on the board, without having to be taken off, spread on tulle gras, and separately transferred.

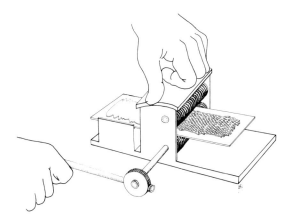

Fig. 2.6 Modified skin-meshing technique. The plastic board is initially cut across and the skin placed onto adjacent squares. This technique gives parallel perforations which are not staggered, and do not allow the skin to stretch. Haematoma is therefore prevented, as the meshes allow release of oozing from the recipient bed, and the cosmetic result of the graft is better than that obtained with expanded meshed skin graft.

skin may be quite satisfactorily perforated by hand using a #15 scalpel blade, but Browne (1988) has shown that a regular pattern of non-expandable perforations is achieved if the graft is placed on a cut-up meshboard which is fed into the roller blade at 90° to the normal orientation (Fig. 2.6). This pattern of perforations heals well and produces a satisfactory cosmetic result.

Although thick split-skin grafts, or full-thickness grafts, have been meshed to enhance skin-graft take, meshing may leave unfavourable scars. Pigmented skin may likewise heal with very prominent scars if meshing is carried out. Even when full-thickness or thick split-thickness grafts are used, scar contracture may occur at the margins of the graft. Where possible, skin-graft cover of larger areas should be provided in anatomical units, so that the marginal scars are most favourably placed.

GRAFT THICKNESS

It was long ago realized that nutritional requirements are much reduced in thin skin grafts, which therefore take more readily. Full-thickness grafts have a less certain initial course because their nutritional demands are much greater. This was typified in one of the earliest descriptions of thick skin grafting (Bünger 1823) when skin cut from the outer thigh was applied to the freshened stump of a nose. The case was reported as a success, although a large part of the graft became necrotic.

Skin grafts applied to the hand may be partial thickness, full thickness, or composite (in that the graft contains subcutaneous or other tissue). Thin skin grafts are usually less than 0.010 in thick, while the most commonly used medium-thickness grafts contain more dermis and are in the region of 0.010–0.022 in thick. The actual thickness of 'full thickness' and 'partial thickness' grafts is, however, variable, depending on the donor site. Skin thickness varies with age, increasing through childhood until the fourth decade, when it progressively thins again (Southwood 1955). Skin is thickest on the soles of the feet, and thinnest on the eyelids. Most of the thickness difference is due

to the epidermis – Southwood reported that the thickness of the epidermis of the sole is 0.53 mm–1.38 mm, and that on the lateral thigh is 0.03 mm–0.08 mm. The dermis of the sole is 0.87–1.80 mm thick, and on the lateral thigh it is 0.56–1.80 mm thick. Equivalent areas of skin are thicker in males than in females. Care should therefore be exercised in cutting skin grafts in small children, elderly patients, and those who may have thin skin or another reason, such as systemic steroid therapy.

INDICATIONS FOR SKIN GRAFTS

To achieve temporary cover

To close an open wound and prevent infection, hasten initial healing, and prevent exposure of underlying structures.

The protective and barrier functions of skin depend on an intact epidermis, and these properties are effective as soon as the skin containing intact epidermis is applied. Thin skin grafts have a low nutritional requirement, and therefore a much better ability to take, even when the recipient bed is imperfect, at the time of primary surgery. The grafts are applied as 'biological dressings' and will often take, to seal and protect a raw surface until definitive surgery is carried out later.

Thin grafts may be used in this way on wounds which are to be surgically reviewed again within a short time; to achieve immediate cover of defects in the hand which will not close due to oedema, but where there has been no actual skin loss, (e.g. following fasciotomies); or over the pedicle of a free vascularized flap or a replanted digit, where tension caused by flap closure would risk vascular occlusion. In these situations the grafts may be meshed to allow the escape of exudate which would otherwise raise the skin from its bed. Once adhesion has occurred the diamond-shaped meshwork defects will close rapidly, especially if the skin is meshed but not expanded. The longer-term disadvantages of thin skin cover can be ignored when skin is being used in this way.

For definitive cover

To provide permanent skin replacement which is

supple, sensate and durable, or to resurface areas of scarring or contracture.

The lack of dermis makes thin skin grafts inappropriate for permanent cover, as they may contract and wrinkle, become abnormally pigmented, and are poorly resistant to trauma. There are, however, a few situations when the contracture of thin (less than 0.010 in thick) grafts may be an advantage, when they are applied to small defects in the knowledge that contracture will occur and pull in normal, sensate skin. This situation is found with wounds of the terminal finger pulps.

Wolfe grafts are indicated because they provide good quality of cover, characterized by supple, sensate skin with no contracture within the graft and, in children, the ability to grow. The decision to use a Wolfe graft will often depend on the adequacy of the recipient bed and the size of the graft required, as the donor site will itself require surgical closure. Wolfe grafts, or at any rate thick split-thickness grafts, will always be preferred for clean surgical defects such as the donor site of a cross-finger flap. It may be desirable in some instances to achieve initial cover with a thin graft and then to provide definitive cover at a secondary procedure when conditions for graft take are more favourable.

In avulsion injuries, it is occasionally possible to preserve the specialized palmar skin as a full-thickness graft, but often the skin itself is damaged, especially on the dorsal surface.

Composite grafts have been advocated by some authors, especially in children (Rees 1960). The replaced avulsed skin and soft tissue of the finger pulp will occasionally take, and if the graft is successful will achieve excellent reconstruction (Douglas 1959). However, it is often found that the fragment does not revascularize. If it remains dry it should be left against the fingertip as a biological dressing, and in children the underlying defect will often heal by cicatrization and epithelialization. Other authors have advocated immediate composite grafting using a segment of toe pulp (McCash 1959). The toe defect requires surgical closure and the take of such non-vascularized toe-to-hand grafts is uncertain.

Composite skin graft may be made to take more reliably if the skin fragment is revascularized by vascular reanastomosis of a vein included with the skin, either to veins or to an artery at one end and a vein at the other (Yoshimura et al 1987; see also Chapter 11). This unconventional revascularization (either pure venous drainage, or the creation of an arteriovenous fistula) effectively converts the graft to a vascularized flap.

PREREQUISITES FOR SKIN GRAFTING

Skin grafts of any thickness may be made to take. All require firm and even contact with a well-vascularized base. The continuing viability of a skin graft depends on the nutritional and metabolic needs of the graft being met, so that revascularization can progress before cell death occurs. In wounds undergoing immediate surgery, all obviously dead or damaged tissue is excised, leaving behind a healthy, bleeding layer on which skin may be placed. In the patient undergoing later surgery, viability will have been established by the presence of a carpet of dry, bright-red granulations which bleed freely on abrasion with a moist swab.

Large areas of cortical bone, tendon, cartilage and joint capsules will not themselves support a graft, but parts of a graft placed over small areas of avascular tissue will derive enough nutrition from collateral circulation within the graft to survive, provided the rest of the bed is vascular. This phenomenon has been termed 'bridging' (McGregor 1965). Larger avascular areas may be rendered able to take a skin graft by the use of pedicled flaps. The use of skin flaps in this specific situation differs from their normal role in reconstruction because it is the skin graft which becomes the permanent skin surface, rather than the skin of the flap.

One-stage local flap cover with vascular tissue and immediate grafting

When the area of avascular tissue is small, it is often possible to mobilize and bring in adjacent soft tissue (e.g. paratenon over tendon; fat or muscle over cortical bone), to provide a vascular recipient bed for a skin graft.

Staged flap cover, return and secondary skin grafting

The principle of the 'crane flap' was described by Millard (1969). In situations where a skin graft cannot be applied primarily because the area is large and partially avascular (such as in large shaved or skiving injuries of the dorsal hand where multiple segments of bone are exposed), a thick pedicled flap may be brought in to cover the defect. This is split horizontally after a period of inset, when the subcutaneous tissue in the deeper layers of the flap has become adherent to the base of the defect. The recipient site is now covered with a layer of vascularized tissue which has bridged over the avascular segments, and skin grafting is now possible. The skin element of the flap, likened by Millard to a crane working at the dockside, has carried across a load (of subcutaneous tissue), is dissected free and swung back to its base. A skin graft on the resulting thin but vascular base will conform more closely to the contours of the hand than the full thickness of a large flap, and will provide satisfactory permanent replacement for the skin of the hand.

Other situations where flaps are initially applied to create a vascular bed are:

1. The dorsum of the finger. Cover may be achieved with a pedicled flap of subcutaneous tissue (Atasoy 1982) which is turned into the defect and immediately grafted (Fig. 2.7). The skin of the donor site is replaced so that there is no donor site defect. Alternatively, a reversed dermis cross-finger flap may be created, where the surface of the flap is deepithelialized and the whole flap turned into the defect. The subcutaneous surface of the flap, which is now outermost, is immediately skin-grafted, as is the donor site defect (Pakiam 1978). The pedicle of the flap is divided at 2 weeks.

2. The finger tip. In many instances it is possible to mobilize adjacent fat to cover small areas of exposed bone, so that the defect can be skin-grafted. As an alternative to the use of a local flap, a distant flap may be applied to the fingertip, with

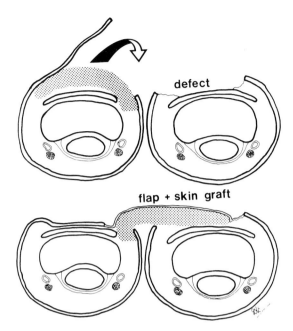

Fig. 2.7 The subcutaneous pedicled flap technique (Atasoy 1982). A superficial skin flap based on the opposite side of the donor digit is raised to gain access to the subcutis, and a subcutaneous flap, based on the same side of the donor digit as the recipient, is swung over and used to cover the defect in the adjacent finger with an immediate skin graft. The thin skin flap in the donor digit is replaced to obviate a full-thickness secondary defect.

the deepithelialized surface facing against the depths of the defect (Morris 1981; see also Chapter 5). It is claimed that the rich dermal vasculature exposed by deepithelialization and which is placed against the base of the defect, enables a more rapid revascularization than does a conventional flap. After a week the flap is divided, the excess fat is trimmed to prevent bulkiness and the skin is grafted.

3. Other finger and hand sites. One-stage random-pattern flaps (Thatte et al 1982) may be created at almost any site in the dorsal or volar hand, provided that sufficient uninjured tissue remains adjacent to the defect to enable a deepithelialized flap to be turned over and skin grafted as a one-stage procedure. Such flaps can be of random vascular supply, may be orientated in any direction, and have been successfully used for recreating web spaces and resurfacing the volar aspect of the finger. However, a large area of skin graft is necessary, to cover both the flap donor site

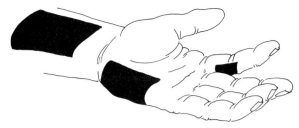

Fig. 2.8 Donor sites for split-thickness skin grafts in the hand and forearm.

and the defect, and as with all reversed dermis techniques there is sacrifice of the specialized functions of the skin contained within the flap when the epidermis is removed and the flap is turned downwards into the defect.

CHOICE OF SKIN-GRAFT DONOR SITES

Partial thickness

Larger areas of skin are taken from the arm or leg, using a graft knife. The forearm is often used, but with larger areas it has the disadvantage that the donor site may remain conspicuous and is difficult to conceal. Thicker skin, (at three-quarters skin thickness, 0.020–0.024 in) may be harvested using a drum dermatome. This provides many of the advantages of a full-thickness skin graft, while the donor site is able to heal (Padgett 1942). The lower abdomen may be used as a donor site and each sheet of graft obtained will provide seamless cover for one surface of the hand.

Most requirements are for smaller areas of skin, which may conveniently be obtained locally in the hand and forearm (Fig. 2.8). In many instances the graft may be cut freehand using a scalpel, such

as the disposable Gillette 'A' blade, or a #10 or #22 blade on a Bard–Parker handle; or a small skin-graft knife such as Silver's (Fig. 2.9), the Weck, Goulian or small Rosenberg knives, which use disposable blades. A special large scalpel blade is available to fit standard Bard–Parker handles (Henderson 1982), and the graft is cut with the unguarded blade. However, a strip of skin over 1 in wide and 0.014 in thick, and as long as desired (depending on the chosen donor site) may be obtained using a standard Schick injector razor (Snow 1968; Fig. 2.10). A freshly sterilized disposable blade is inserted into the razor, which is then held between thumb and forefinger to produce a graft of consistent thickness, protected by the razor's own guard. Other patterns of domestic razor where the blade is supported in its midportion by struts are not suitable.

The freehand methods of split-skin grafting require a steady hand: small areas such as the hypothenar prominence (Fig. 2.11), or the proximal phalanx of a finger may be tensed by the surgeon himself between the forefinger and thumb of the opposite hand whilst the graft is being cut, but assistance in tensing the skin is invaluable if anything other than a small area of graft is to be obtained. It is helpful to infiltrate the skin with saline or local anaesthetic solution in the subdermal plane to make cutting easier.

A dressing is applied to the raw donor site to promote epithelialization: traditionally a non-adherent paraffin gauze sheet with an absorbent backing, but alternatively a moisture-retaining dressing such as polyurethane film (Birdsell et al 1978), hydrophilic gel sheet, or calcium alginate (Attwood 1989).

Local sites

Available donor sites in the hand for split-thickness grafts (Fig. 2.8) are: the hypothenar border of the hand (Patton 1969); the side of the proximal phalanx (Chase 1984); the volar aspect of the forearm (Xavier & Lamb 1974); the palm (Worthen 1973). These donor sites are readily accessible without the need to prepare another area. If surgery is being carried out under regional anaesthesia, the donor site will already be anaesthetized. The palm provides pale, keratinized skin,

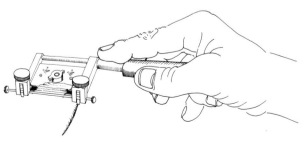

Fig. 2.9 An adjustable small dermatome designed to take safety razor blades (Silver's knife).

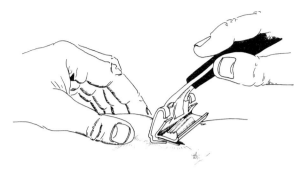

Fig. 2.10 Taking a skin graft with an unmodified Schick injector razor (Snow 1968). A continuous ribbon of skin may be taken.

which is the best replacement for other volar skin defects. In patients with coloured skins, the use of the palm avoids the placement of pigmented skin in a normally pale area.

The volar aspect of the forearm is hairless and also readily accessible. In a review of one series (Xavier & Lamb 1974) no patients suffered donor-site hypertrophy or hyperpigmentation, but hypopigmentation was significant in 60% of patients, some of whom felt that they were stigmatized.

Distant sites

Thick split-thickness grafts from the plantar surface (Fig. 2.12) provide an excellent functional and cosmetic replacement for palmar defects

(Namba et al 1977). Plantar skin shares many characteristics with palmar skin and provides an ideal substitute for it. However, the harvesting of a full-thickness plantar skin graft (Webster 1955) creates a donor-site defect which itself requires skin grafting. The plantar skin is heavily keratinized, and thin skin grafts from this area carry a significant failure rate (LeWorthy 1963). The thickness of the plantar skin means that the measured thickness of grafts from the sole does not necessarily correlate with the 'anatomical thickness', so that an apparently very thick graft is necessary to be certain of including sufficient dermis to prevent graft contracture in the recipient site (Nakamura et al 1984). When a graft is taken at the level of the reticular dermis, punctate areas of fat are visible but healing is nonetheless satisfactory, probably because of the richness of epithelial structures – for example, six times the number of sweat ducts are present in the sole as in the thigh (Szabo 1967). The skin from both soles is available and will resurface a complete palm. Donor-site scar hypertrophy occurs in 25% of patients (Nakamura et al 1984), but causes no functional problems, discomfort or other symptoms.

As a refinement of technique it is possible to take the graft from the instep to include both lateral (pigmented) and plantar (non-pigmented) skin, so that grafts to the finger webs may be appropriately pigmented in coloured patients;

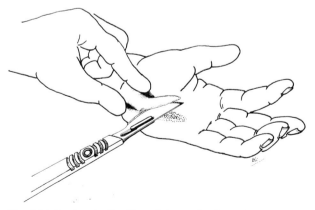

Fig. 2.11 Freehand split-skin graft harvesting from the hypothenar eminence. Either a large standard scalpel blade may be used, or a special skin graft blade (Henderson 1982) mounted on a standard scalpel handle. Prior infiltration of local anaesthetic makes the donor site firm, and also gives postoperative analgesia.

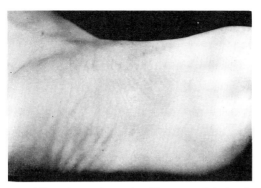

Fig. 2.12 The sole as a donor site. The non-weight-bearing area which may be taken is marked by skin creases when the foot is plantar flexed. The skin is distended with a local anaesthetic injection, tensed, and the skin harvested whilst an assistant holds the foot dorsiflexed. A refinement of the technique is to take an initial very thin epidermal graft, then to take a thicker partial thickness graft including the remaining epidermis and as much dermis as required, and then to cover the raw area with the initial epidermal graft. This secures haemostasis and relieves donor-site pain. The epidermis may be hand-perforated to enhance take.

(Ward & Ecclestone 1985; Fig. 2.13, 2.14), as well as providing like replacement for both dorsal and volar skin. However, these authors noted significant donor-site morbidity in adult patients although children had no problems with pain, delayed healing, or difficulty with gait.

Full thickness

Several useful donor sites have been described. The choice for larger areas is limited to the groin, or areas of the torso, which present donor sites

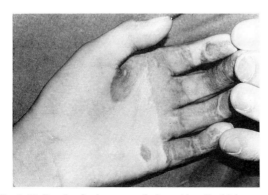

Fig. 2.13 Result of palmar resurfacing with split-thickness skin from the thigh in an Indian child. In addition to the unsightly pigmentation, there has been flexion contracture of the fingers.

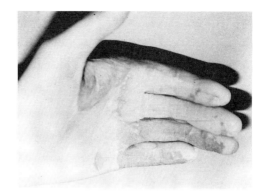

Fig. 2.14 After excision of pigmented skin graft, and partial resurfacing of the pigmented area using thick plantar skin grafts. One sole was used, and was subsequently, reharvested for the remaining pigmented area. The colour and texture of the palmar skin were improved by use of the similar plantar skin.

from which a large area of skin may be taken with primary closure of the donor defect. However, the colour match of groin skin is often imperfect and the cosmetic result may be marred by hair growth. Skin from the torso is thicker and of coarser texture than that normally present on the hand.

There has been much interest in techniques which enhance the take of full-thickness skin grafts. Tsukuda (1980) has described the technique for harvesting a full-thickness skin graft in which the subcutaneous vascular network is intentionally preserved by a very conservative excision

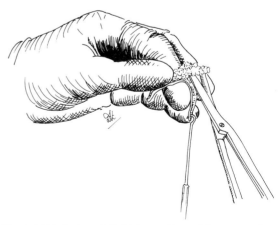

Fig. 2.15 Defatting a full-thickness skin graft is more easily achieved if the graft is kept under tension over the operator's finger. Care should be taken not to thin the graft too radically, as it is desired that the subcutaneous vascular network should be preserved.

of subcutaneous fat (Fig. 2.15). He believes that the preserved subcutaneous vascular network is immediately available for anastomosis with vessels in the recipient site, and suggests that the preservation of areolar tissues in the plane below the skin prevents any tendency to postoperative wrinkling, contracture or scar formation. This belief is in keeping with the electron microscopic studies of Okada (1986), referred to above (see page 13).

Smaller areas of full-thickness skin graft are readily obtained from areas of lax skin in the hand (Fig. 2.16): an ellipse with a width of 2 cm and a length of 6 cm may be taken from the hypothenar area in adult patients (Schenck & Cheema 1984) and provides a good quality sensate skin graft, with an acceptable donor-site defect. A slightly smaller curved ellipse (3 cm × 1.5 cm) of full-thickness skin is available from the palm, being taken from the radial side of the thenar crease (Mack et al 1981). This donor site can be uncomfortable, and splintage of the hand is advisable in the early stages of healing. Smaller Wolfe grafts may be taken from the sides of proximal phalanges with direct closure of the donor site.

Smaller areas of full-thickness skin may be obtained from skin crease areas at the wrist and brachial fossa, or from the forearm. There will inevitably be considerable distracting force across the scar at the donor site, which should be securely closed, e.g. with subcuticular monofilament sutures. Full-thickness skin may be taken from the supraclavicular area, (where the donor scar will be conspicuous), or the inframammary crease in women. The postauricular donor site gives a concealed scar but the thinness, texture and colour of skin from this area are not always a good match with the hand. Other donor sites may

be used but will require skin grafting themselves, e.g. the dorsum of the foot.

It is also possible to transfer full-thickness skin as a free non-vascularized graft, whilst preserving a sensory nerve which allows movement of the skin to the recipient site (e.g. from the dorsum of the index finger to the thumb, preserving the superficial terminal branch of the radial nerve. This technique is more often performed as a cross-finger flap.). Several donor sites for sensate, vascularized free flaps have been described from the foot, but it is also possible to perform a transfer with small areas of skin taken as an ordinary Wolfe graft (Lister 1969). The sensation recovered after reanastomosis of the nerve taken with the Wolfe graft may not achieve normality, even though the technique offers theoretical advantages over the random reinnervation of a Wolfe graft by mere ingrowth of nerve ends from the graft bed and margins. A comparative study has not yet been reported.

SKIN GRAFTS IN NAILBED RECONSTRUCTION

Careful primary repair of the nailbed at the time of injury will often produce an acceptable result in terms of nail growth, adhesion and appearance. The avulsed nailbed represents highly specialized tissue which it is impossible to match perfectly, and the fragment of tissue (with the nail attached) should be replaced as a composite graft (Zook 1985).

The nailbed presents a particular problem, however, following severe tissue destruction or inadequate primary surgery. Nail regrowth will not occur if the germinal matrix is damaged, and there will be no nail adhesion (even if growth occurs) if the nailbed or sterile matrix is scarred or ablated.

Reconstruction of the sterile matrix may be either functional or (in cases where the germinal matrix is also affected) purely cosmetic. Reconstruction of the nailbed, preserving the adhesion of the nail, may be achieved with no donor-site morbidity, using a split-thickness nailbed graft from another digit (Shepard 1983). It has also been found that a reversed dermal graft sutured deepithelialized side down into a nailbed defect

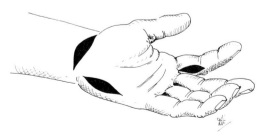

Fig. 2.16 Possible full-thickness skin-graft donor sites in the hand and forearm. These donor sites require direct closure and should therefore be small enough to be sutured.

can achieve satisfactory reconstruction (Clayburgh et al 1983). An alternative technique is to use a full-thickness graft of nailbed from a little toe (Saito 1983) with sacrifice of the donor nail. The germinal matrix is removed from the donor toe to prevent donor-site problems, and may be used to provide additional length for the sterile matrix in the recipient finger. Normal nail adhesion is obtained.

Badly deformed nails or areas of post-traumatic scarring may be grafted with thick split-thickness graft to simulate the appearance of a nail. In the nail pouch technique (Buncke & Gonzalez 1962) the skin graft is wrapped around a stent, implanted, and the soft tissues are later trimmed to create a flat bed and a proximal pocket which will accept a nail prosthesis, fixed by adhesive tape.

SKIN GRAFTS IN BURNS MANAGEMENT
(See also Chapter 16)

Burns of the hand create many difficulties in assessment and treatment. Although restoration of skin cover is important, there are other priorities in the early management of the burned hand. Thermal burns may result in complete circumferential areas of skin destruction with a resulting tight eschar that threatens vascular perfusion – as in all hand injuries the preservation of blood supply takes precedence over the restoration of skin cover. There is always attendant oedema which will result in finger stiffness if inadequately managed by splintage and exercise.

It may not be possible to be certain of the depth of tissue destruction on initial examination. Other forms of burn injury may create smaller areas of deep skin loss: immediate excision of electrical burns may allow primary reconstruction with skin grafts, though debridement of deeply damaged tissues may expose an avascular base, or vital structures such as repaired nerves or arteries which will require flap repair rather than a skin graft.

Following a burn the skin may have lost its structural integrity, and attempts should be made to prevent bacterial infection (as opposed to bacterial colonization of the burned skin surface, which is inevitable). The barrier functions of skin

can be restored by grafting, and early tangential excision and split-skin grafting (Janzekovic 1970) have many exponents. It has, however, been argued that early excision of partial thickness burns of the hand may lead to viable tissue being discarded, and on late comparison of hand burns which had healed following conservative treatment, and those treated by early excision and skin grafting, there was no eventual functional difference (Salisbury & Wright 1982).

Split-thickness skin grafting is, however, the mainstay of the immediate management of the hand burn. Meshed grafts may be preferred, but should be used with a full understanding of their limitations. Bailey (1986, personal communication) has suggested the following practical schema for the role of skin grafting in the management of hand burns:

1. Obvious superficial burns
    small – exposure
    large – occlusive dressing
    whole hand – plastic bag
2. Obvious full-thickness burns
    small – immediate excision and grafting
    extensive (usually associated with other areas of burn) – escharotomy, dressings, eventual grafting
3. Mixed-thickness burns
    escharotomy if needed, dressings, then tangential excision and skin grafting.

At a later stage skin grafts are used to correct skin and joint contractures, and it may be elected to resurface areas initially closed with thinner, meshed skin grafts. At this stage the wound is of established vascularity, there is no infection or oedema, and the conditions favour the take of thick skin grafts, so that better quality skin cover may be obtained.

Patients with hand burns alone will have adequate autogenous skin graft available for the reconstruction and restoration of an intact barrier of grafted skin. However, patients with large areas of burn may lack adequate donor skin for complete cover of the entire burn wound, including the hands. Under these circumstances treatment may be carried out using biological dressings (such as porcine or bovine heterografts, cryopreserved cadaver allografts, or amniotic membrane), or synthetic membranes (such as plastic film, laminated polyurethane foam, silicone polymer membrane, or peptide-bonded silicone/nylon membrane). It must be emphasized that the synthetic materials provide only temporary cover, and even the 'permanent' cover provided by the use of cultured dermal autografts or allografts will be much less satisfactory than a carefully chosen and applied skin graft, had the donor sites been available. There is current interest in comminuted skin as a replacement for split-thickness sheet grafts, but the techniques and long-term results have yet to be fully evaluated.

COMPLICATIONS OF SKIN GRAFTS

Browne (1986) pointed out that conditions which require the replacement of skin coverage are those in which potential wound problems exist, and that unsatisfactory results may sometimes be the inevitable consequence of those conditions. However, the most commonly found complications may be classified as being due to:

1. Wound problems
   Due to grafting on an inadequately prepared or unsuitable bed
   – avascularity
   – infection
2. Graft problems
   Early:
   Failure of take due to inadequate contact between graft/bed
   – inadequate fixation (shearing)
   – haematoma
   Failure of take/graft lysis due to infection
   Late:
   Avoidable scarring/contracture
   – excessively expanded mesh graft
   – graft margins crossing anatomical segments
   Trophic ulceration/trauma
   – graft insensate
   – graft too thin for permanent cover
3. Donor site problems
   Failure to heal
   – infection

– too large for primary closure
– split-thickness graft cut too deep
Inappropriate choice of donor site
– visible scars
– discomfort
  donor scar exposed to trauma
  neuromas
– scar contracture

Other problems such as hypertrophic scarring and abnormal pigmentation should be considered as a side-effect of skin-graft surgery, rather than as avoidable complications.

CONCLUSIONS

Skin grafting in all its forms provides a versatile means for providing many different types of skin cover for hand injuries, enabling the replacement of 'like with like'. It is the most widely applicable and variable surgical technique, and is often the simplest way in which the skin of the hand may be reconstructed. With regard to the size of the hands, there is no limitation in the availability of donor tissue.

Skin-grafting techniques can be precisely tailored to the specific requirements of the recipient area, and indeed it is desirable that the most appropriate donor site should be selected. Grafting techniques may be used for temporary or permanent cover, and in association with flap techniques, or to immediately reconstruct the secondary defects of flaps used in primary hand reconstruction.

Many new flap techniques are now available for restoring skin cover to the hand. The hand surgeon should, however, remember that skin grafts are quick and simple to harvest and inset, and will provide reliable skin cover when used appropriately to resurface hand defects. Even when considering those series which enthusiastically advocate the primary use of flaps for skin cover, it may often be seen that carefully applied skin-grafting techniques have provided the largest group of patients with single-stage reconstruction and the lowest long-term complication rates.

REFERENCES

Atasoy E 1982 Reversed cross-finger subcutaneous flap. Journal of Hand Surgery 7: 481

Attwood A I 1989 Calcium alginate accelerates skin graft donor site healing. British Journal of Plastic Surgery 42: 373

Barron J N 1970 The structure and function of the skin of the hand. Hand 2: 93

Bert P 1863 La greffe animale. Baillière, Paris

Birdsell, D C, Hein K S, Lindsay R L 1978 The theoretically ideal donor site dressing. Annals of Plastic Surgery 2: 535

Browne E Z 1986 Complications of skin grafts and pedicle flaps. Hand Clinics 2: 353

Browne E Z 1988 Mesh grafting. In: Green D P (ed) Operative Hand Surgery Vol 3, Churchill Livingstone, New York, p 1826

Buncke H J Jr, Gonzalez R I 1962 Fingernail reconstruction. Plastic and Reconstructive Surgery 30: 452

Bünger H C 1823 Gelungener Versuch einer Nasenbildung aus einem völlig getrennten Hautstück aus dem Beine. Gr. u. Augenh. Bd 4: 569

Burd D A R 1984 The pressure button: a refinement of the traditional 'tie over' dressing. British Journal of Plastic Surgery 37: 127

Byars L T 1942 Free full thickness skin grafts: principles involved and technique of application. Surgery Gynecology and Obstetrics 75: 8

Chase R A 1984 Skin grafting. In: Atlas of Hand Surgery, Vol 2, W.B. Saunders, Philadelphia, p 18

Clayburgh R H, Wood M B, Cooney W P 1983 Nail bed reconstruction by reverse dermal grafts. Journal of Hand Surgery 8: 594

Conway H 1939 Sweating function of transplanted skin. Surgery Gynecology and Obstetrics 69: 756

Cooper A 1827 The lectures of Sir Astley Cooper Bart FRS on the principles and practice of surgery, with additional notes and cases by Frederick Tyrrell. Lecture XXXVI, Volume 3. Underwood, London, p 149

Davis J S, Kitlowski E A 1931 The immediate contraction of skin grafts and its cause. Archives of Surgery 23: 954

Douglas B 1959 Successful replacement of completely avulsed portions of fingers as composite grafts. Plastic and Reconstructive Surgery 23: 213

Fitzgerald M J T, Martin F, Paletta F X 1967 Innervation of skin grafts. Surgery Gynecology and Obstetrics 124: 808

Fitzpatrick T P, Szabo G 1959 The melanocyte: cytology and cytochemistry. Journal of Investigative Dermatology 32: 197

Henderson H P 1982 A simple skin graft blade for use on a scalpel handle. British Journal of Plastic Surgery 35: 394

Hinshaw J R, Miller E R 1965 Histology of healing split-thickness, full-thickness autogenous skin grafts and donor sites. Archives of Surgery 91: 658

Janzekovic A 1970 A new concept in the early excision and immediate grafting of burns. Journal of Trauma 10: 1103

LeWorthy G W 1963 Sole skin as a donor site to replace palmar skin. Plastic and Reconstructive Surgery 32: 30

Lister G D 1969 Use of an innervated skin graft to provide sensation to the reconstructed heel. British Journal of Plastic Surgery 22: 143

McCash C R 1959 Toe pulp free grafts in finger-tip repair. British Journal of Plastic Surgery 11: 322

McGregor I A 1965 Fundamental techniques of plastic surgery, 3rd edn E & S Livingstone, Edinburgh, p 53–96

McGregor I A 1970 Degloving injuries. Hand 2: 130

Mack G R, Neviaser R J, Wilson J N 1981 Free palmar skin grafts for resurfacing digital defects. Journal of Hand Surgery 6: 565

Magnier 1874 Epidermic grafts to avoid the contracture of a large avulsion injury of the back of the hand. Gazette Médicale Paris, 4 s, 3: 253

Medawar P B 1944 The behaviour and fate of skin autografts and skin homografts in rabbits. Journal of Anatomy 78: 176

Medawar P B 1945 The experimental study of skin grafts. British Medical Bulletin 3: 79

Millard D R 1969 The crane principle for the transport of subcutaneous tissue. Plastic and Reconstructive Surgery 43: 451

Morris A McG 1981 Rapid skin cover in hand injuries using the reverse-dermis flap. British Journal of Plastic Surgery 34: 194

Nakamura K, Namba K, Tsuchida H 1984 A retrospective study of thick split thickness plantar skin grafts to resurface the palm. Annals of Plastic Surgery 12: 508

Namba K, Tsuchida H, Nakamura K 1977 Split-skin grafts from the hairless area for resurfacing of palmar surface of the hand. Japan Journal of Plastic and Reconstructive Surgery 20: 584

Okada T 1986 Revascularisation of free full thickness skin grafts in rabbits: a scanning electron microscope study of microvascular casts. British Journal of Plastic Surgery 39: 183

Ollier L X E L 1872 Cutaneous or autoplastic grafts. Bulletin de e'Académie Médicale, Paris, 2 s, 1: 243

Padgett E C 1942 Skin grafting. Charles C. Thomas, Springfield, Illinois, pp 34–68

Pakiam A I 1978 The reversed dermis flap. British Journal of Plastic Surgery 31: 131

Patton H S 1969 Split skin graft from hypothenar area for fingertip avulsions. Plastic and Reconstructive Surgery 15: 426

Petry J J, Wortham K A 1986 Contraction and growth of wounds covered by meshed and non-meshed split thickness grafts. British Journal of Plastic Surgery 39: 478

Ponten B 1960 Grafted skin: observations on innervation and other qualities. Acta Chirurgia Scandinavica (Suppl.) 257: 1

Ragnell A 1953 The secondary contracting tendency of free skin grafts. British Journal of Plastic Surgery 5: 6

Rees T D 1960 The transfer of composite grafts of skin and fat: a clinical study. Plastic and Reconstructive Surgery 25: 556

Reverdin 1869 Epidermic grafts. Bulletin Société imperiale de Chirurgie, Paris, 2 s, 10: 493; 511

Rudolph R, Klein L 1973 Healing processes in skin grafts. Surgery Gynecology and Obstetrics 136: 641

Saito H, Suzuki Y, Fujino K, Tajima T 1983 Free nail bed graft for treatment of nail bed injuries of the hand. Journal of Hand Surgery 8: 171

Salisbury R E, Wright P 1982 Evaluation of early excision of dorsal burns of the hand. Plastic and Reconstructive Surgery 69: 670

Schenck R R, Cheema T A 1984 Hypothenar skin grafts for fingertip reconstruction. Journal of Hand Surgery 9A: 750

Shepard G H 1983 Treatment of nail bed avulsions with split thickness nail bed grafts. Journal of Hand Surgery 8: 49

Šmahel J 1965 Development of hematomas under a free skin autograft. Plastic and Reconstructive Surgery 35: 207

Šmahel J 1977 The healing of skin grafts. Clinics in Plastic Surgery 4: 3 409

Snow J W 1968 Safety razor dermatome. Plastic and Reconstructive Surgery 41: 184

Southwood W F W 1955 The thickness of the skin. Plastic and Reconstructive Surgery 15: 423

Szabo G 1967 The regional anatomy of the human integument with special reference to the distribution of hair follicles, sweat glands, and melanocytes. Philosophical Transactions of the Royal Society, London (Biol) 252: 447

Tanner J C, Vandeput J, Olley J F 1964 The mesh skin graft. Plastic and Reconstructive Surgery 34: 287

Thatte R, Gopalakrishna A, Prasad S 1982 The use of de-epithelialised 'turn-over' flaps in the hand. British Journal of Plastic Surgery 35: 293

Thiersch C 1886 Über Hautverplanzung. Verhandluno deutscher Gesellschaft Chirurgie 15: 17

Tsukuda S 1980 Transfer of free skin grafts with a preserved subcutaneous vascular network. Annals of Plastic Surgery 4: 500

Ward C M, Ecclestone J 1985 The use of split thickness grafts from the instep in paediatric hand surgery. Journal of Hand Surgery 10B: 185

Waris T 1978 Reinnervation of free skin autografts in the rat. Scandinavian Journal of Plastic and Reconstructive Surgery 12: 85

Waris T, Rechardt L, Kyösola, K Y 1983 Reinnervation of human skin grafts: a histochemical study. Plastic and Reconstructive Surgery 72: 439

Waris T Åstrand K, Hämäläinen H, Piironen J, Valtimo J, Järvilehto T 1989 Regeneration of cold, warm and heat pain sensibility in human skin grafts. British Journal of Plastic Surgery 42: 576

Webster J P 1955 Skin grafts for hairless areas of the hands and feet. Plastic and Reconstructive Surgery 15: 83

Wolfe J R 1875 A new method of performing plastic operations. British Medical Journal 2: 360

Wood-Jones F 1942 Principles of anatomy as seen in the hand. 2nd edn. Baillière Tindall & Cox, London

Worthen E F 1973 The palmar split skin graft. British Journal of Plastic Surgery 26: 408

Xavier T S, Lamb D W 1974 The forearm as donor site for split skin grafts. Hand 6: 243

Yoshimura M, Shimada T, Imura S, Shimamura K, Yamauchi S 1987 The venous skin graft method for repairing defects of the fingers. Plastic and Reconstructive Surgery 79: 243

Zook E G 1985 Nail bed injuries. Hand Clinics 1: 701

3

Local skin flaps in the hand

The hand is the prime means by which man can modify his environment, and it has therefore evolved into a highly specialized organ. The skin, acting as an interface between the delicate sensitive structures of the hand and the outside world, has perfected its roles of sensation and protection whilst simultaneously allowing mobility.

The volar surface of the hand is covered by tough, yet highly sensate, hairless skin tightly bound to the underlying bone. This skin lacks sebaceous glands and has multiple fine ridges to facilitate grip. The dorsal surface has evolved the nail, a keratin appendage, to help support and stabilize the tip pulp and amplify the sensation of this most sensitive part of the digit. The remainder of the dorsal surface has mobile, thin distensible skin, which permits the mobility of the underlying tendons, ranging from hyperextension to a clenched fist.

The hand is often injured and frequently sustains skin loss because of its vital role in the domestic and industrial environments. The problem of skin replacement faces the hand surgeon after the correction of congenital deformities, ablation of skin tumours affecting the hand, and after correction of Dupuytren's contracture. The necessity for rapid skin replacement and effective primary healing of the hand is firstly to reduce the scar, following the production of granulation tissue, which restricts the suppleness of the hand; secondly to reduce the time that an open wound exposes the hand to the entry of infective organisms, and thirdly to preserve the viability of underlying vulnerable structures. Other reasons for skin replacement include the provision of sensation at key points (e.g. fingertips), provision of

durable skin to permit later reconstructive procedures on underlying structures, and finally to prevent contracture formation.

As in any surgical discipline there are several solutions to any given problem. The role of the surgeon is to select the most appropriate technique for a given patient with any particular lesion; the surgeon must therefore assess each patient independently. The age of the patient, handedness, single or multiple digital involvement, the particular digit injured, the patient's occupation and hobbies and preexisting hand and digital trauma or disease all should be assessed in the initial history. The examiner should note the shape of the hand and digits and assess the possibility of using local flaps. The positioning of joints to permit the apposition of digits for cross-finger flap transfer from donor to recipient sites should also be considered.

For the sake of clarity, the hand and digits will be divided into regions and methods of reconstructing skin loss, and the problems specific to each region will be discussed in turn. As the fingertip is an unique area of the finger this will be discussed separately, as will the thumb, which, being the most important digit, must retain maximum length to facilitate opposition.

VOLAR SKIN LOSS

Fingertip injuries (see also Chapter 15)

These can be divided into those with exposed bone and those without. If there is no exposed bone the defect can be dealt with by a skin grafting technique. However, if bone is exposed two

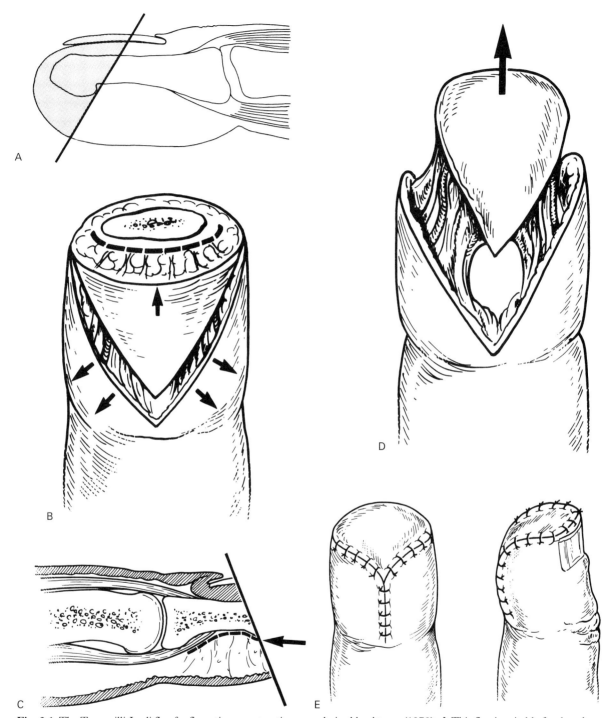

Fig. 3.1 The Tranquilli-Leali flap for fingertip reconstruction, popularized by Atasoy (1970). **A** This flap is suitable for dorsal sloping amputations where more of the volar structures remain than the dorsal structures. **B** The triangular flap is undermined just below the dermis in a proximal direction to allow advancement of the base of the triangle distally. **C** The vertical septae which hold the pulp tissue to the periosteum are then divided. These must be divided above the level of the periosteum, leaving periosteum attached to bone, otherwise the flap will not advance. **D** The flap is then advanced, based on the volar branches of the termination of the neurovascular bundles on either side of the fingertip. **E** The final result with the flap in place and the secondary defect sutured.

factors must be considered: the length of remaining distal phalangeal shaft to support the nailbed, and the slope of the wound edge. If more than half the nailbed and underlying phalanx has been lost, then attempts at nail preservation without nailbed support result in a 'parrot beak' nail which separates from its bed, is cosmetically unsightly and functionally awkward, readily catching on objects and splitting or tearing away further from the bed. Therefore with loss of more than half the nailbed and underlying phalanx, nail ablation is advisable as part of the stump closure technique.

Bone exposed with preservation of half the nailbed

If the nail is to be preserved and if the wound is sloping dorsally or is transverse, then a Tranquilli-Leali V-Y volar advancement flap is appropriate (Tranquilli-Leali 1935; Fig. 3.1). This is a neurovascular island flap advanced on the V-Y principle. Under regional anaesthesia and exsanguination (either limb or digital) the flap is marked and raised as a triangle with its base distal and the apex at the distal interphalangeal (DIP) joint crease (Atasoy et al 1970). The base should only be wide enough to cover the exposed bone, as the wider the base the more obtuse the angle at the apex and the more difficult it is to achieve flap advancement. The skin is incised only through the full thickness of the dermis. This can be easily done by stretching the skin on either side of the intended incision line and cutting until the subcutaneous fat protrudes, under tension, into the wound.

It is vital not to cut deeper than the dermis, as the flap survives on the terminal branches of both digital arteries, which run obliquely from the trifurcation of the digital artery just distal to the DIP joint crease, towards the midline of the pulp. These vessels run in the subdermal plane, so that deepening the skin incision beyond the dermis will place them at risk. The skin is then undermined proximally, again just below the dermis. Now the vertical fibrous septae which bind the skin of the pulp to the underlying distal phalangeal tuft are divided just superficial to the periosteum. As these are divided advancement can be attained. The base of the flap is sutured to the risidual nail stump and at the apex the secondary defect is closed as a V-Y. This is again facilitated by an acute apical angle to the flap triangle. A light dressing is applied to allow continued metacarpophalangeal (MP) and proximal interphalangeal (PIP) joint movement. Sutures should be left for at least 3 weeks or the flap may retract from the nail, exposing the distal bone stump.

The advantages of this technique are that it is a quick, single-staged procedure to obtain an advancement of up to 1 cm, giving sensate skin of reliable vascularity to cover the bone stump without joint immobilization. It can also be skewed obliquely to cover oblique tip loss.

An alternative technique in oblique amputation is the oblique triangular flap described by Venkataswami and Subramanian (1980; Fig. 3.2). In this technique an oblique triangle is marked, with the base equal in width to the amputation site and having one side longer than the other. The shorter straight side of the triangle is in the long axis of the digit dorsal to the neurovascular bundle. The length of the flap depends on the advancement necessary, but is usually 2–2.5 times the base of the triangle, so that sometimes the triangle crosses the joint crease. The flap is raised off the fibrous flexor sheath on the neurovascular bundle, from distal to proximal along the straight dorsal limb of the triangle. At the apex the neurovascular bundle is mobilized. The longer oblique limb is then incised, the fibrous septae being divided under magnification, thus mobilizing the flap. The flap is advanced and sutured to the nail and the secondary defect is closed as a V-Y. The example shown in Fig. 3.2 is a step-advancement island flap as described by Evans and Martin (1988). As the flap moves distally the steps interdigitate in a more distal position.

Other methods available are the lateral V-Y advancement or Kutler flaps. Regrettably in the authors' experience these flaps do not advance easily to cover the bone stump, and would only be recommended in the occasional case where the pattern of skin loss favours this repair technique.

Where skin loss is greater on the volar than on the dorsal surfaces there is little tissue available for local flaps. If the patient is young, and has long slender fingers and supple joints, length can be preserved by either a cross-finger or thenar flap. In patients over about 40 years of age, or those

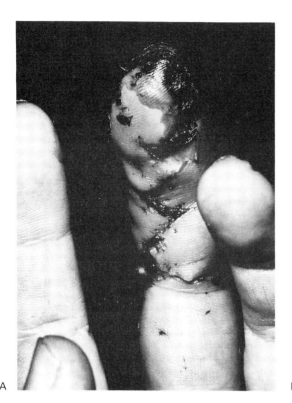

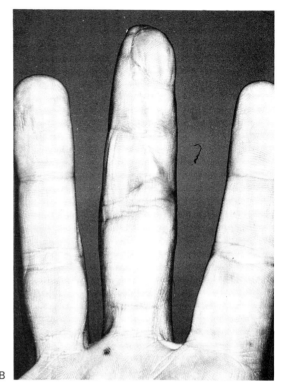

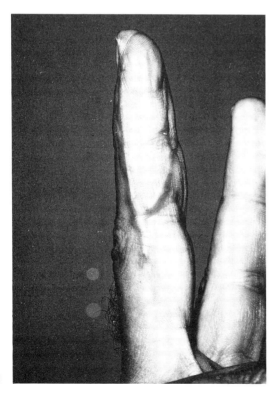

Fig. 3.2 The Venkataswami flap modified by Evans and Martin for fingertip reconstruction. A 49-year-old patient who had sustained a lawnmower injury, amputating the tip of his finger and affecting the radial pulp more than the ulnar side. A step-advancement flap was undertaken. The tip of the flap showed some venous impairment which settled spontaneously. **A** The flap seen approximately 2 weeks after it was raised. **B, C** The flap at 3–4 months. The scars are still red and raised, but did respond to massage and the passage of time.

engaged in heavy work resulting in squat, powerful hands, such flaps are a problem because joint stiffness is a devastating and frequent complication, which can be difficult to correct.

The thenar flap is useful for length preservation in the index or middle fingers of younger patients. Under regional anaesthesia and limb exsanguination a proximally based trapdoor of skin can be raised from the thenar eminence, aligned on the crease at the base of the thumb. The secondary defect can be closed directly to reconstitute the crease, and the flap sutured to the amputated fingertip stump by flexing the MP and PIP joints. The pedicle can be divided at 2 weeks. The advantage of this flap is that it does not scar the adjacent fingers and provides tough, glabrous volar skin.

However, the disadvantages are great – principally that the PIP joint is immobilized in an anatomically compromising position with the collateral ligaments relaxed, so that PIP joint contracture is a real possibility, and this can be difficult to correct once established. Secondly, the donor-site scar can become painful and restrict power grip. Thirdly, the flap is really only suitable for the index fingertip since the middle finger can only be positioned under some tension. Finally, the flap is insensitive when applied to the fingertip, and thus in the presence of a normal middle finger the patient would probably exclude the index from pinch.

A second option for volar sloping skin loss would be a cross-finger flap. These are most commonly aligned transversely, but can also be based either proximally or distally. The donor digit should preferably be either the middle or ring, leaving the dynamic border digits unrestricted by donor sites. The donor site otherwise is selected by the ease with which it can be approximated to the amputation stump. The flap should be raised as the whole dorsal cosmetic unit of the donor digit from midaxial line to midaxial line, and from the extension creases of the PIP joint to the extension creases of the DIP joint for the segment overlying the middle phalanx. The skin over the joints is always preserved to maintain PIP and DIP joint movement unrestricted by dorsal scar (Fig. 3.3).

The whole flap is raised, even if it is larger than required, and the surplus is discarded. This allows the whole cosmetic unit to be replaced by a full-thickness skin graft giving, ultimately, a good cosmetic appearance.

The procedure is performed under regional anaesthesia and limb exsanguination. The positioning of donor and recipient sites is checked and the flap marked. The incision around the margin of the flap is deepened through the dermis. The skin edges are placed under tension, causing the wound edges to part and exposing the subcutaneous veins, which can be cauterized with bipolar diathermy. The wound is then deepened to below the subcutaneous fat, but the paratenon is not disturbed. The flap is elevated in this plane and reflected on its base down to Cleland's ligaments, which may be divided if extra length is required.

The flap is shaped to fit the defect and then the tourniquet is released and fine haemostasis performed. A full-thickness skin graft is harvested from the lateral groin fold, large enough to cover the whole of the secondary defect as well as the undersurface of the flap. This wound is closed directly. Final haemostasis is secured and the skin graft is sutured to the edge of the amputation defect on the side adjacent to the donor digit. This stabilizes one edge of the graft. The flap is sutured over the amputation defect and the skin graft is spread over the pedicle of the flap and the secondary defect of the donor digit, and secured with a tie-over dressing on the other three borders. The fingers are secured with adhesive tape in a position that relieves any tension on the flap, and the hand is splinted in plaster.

If the inset is large, the pedicle could be divided at 2 weeks, but if the inset is small or there is evidence of infection, dehiscence, delayed healing or any other problem, then division should be deferred to 3 weeks. Division should also be performed under regional anaesthesia and limb exsanguination. The pedicle is divided near its base on the donor digit. A triangular area of scar and granulation tissue will be found at the point of reflection from the donor digit and at the beginning of the inset into the recipient site. These triangles must be excised, to allow proper insetting of the pedicle edge of the flap and the base of the pedicle on the donor digit.

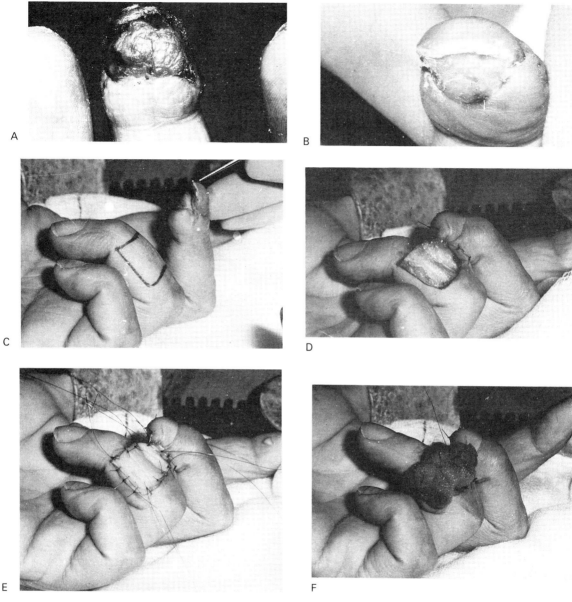

Fig. 3.3 Cross-finger flap reconstruction. This patient had a cross-finger flap performed as part of a revision of an unsatisfactory amputation stump affecting his left middle finger. The tip of the finger had been left to granulate and when the crust was removed the appearance was as in **A**. **B** The nailbed has been released and the defect can be seen from the side. A cross-finger flap was planned and elevated from the adjacent ring finger. It was then applied to the defect as seen in **C** and **D**. **E** A full-thickness skin graft has been applied to the secondary defect on the dorsum of the donor finger. This has been taken from the ulnar border of the hand. **F** A tie-over dressing has been used to maintain the position of the graft. **G** The donor site and the hand at the completion of the procedure.

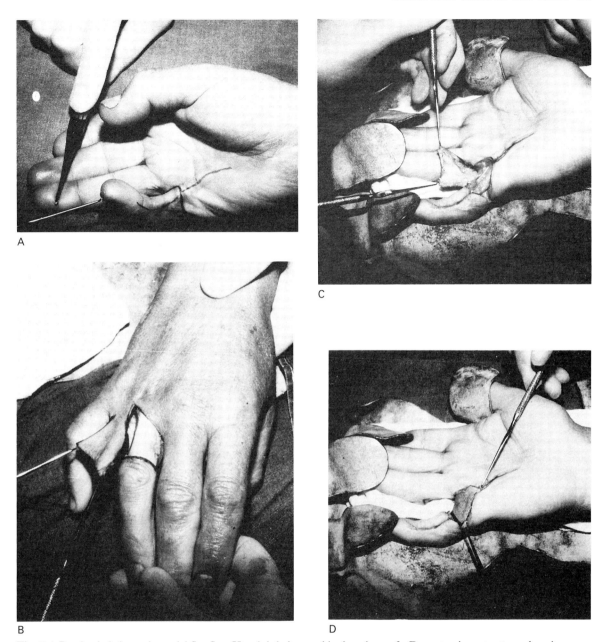

Fig. 3.4 Proximal phalangeal or axial flag flap. Here it is being used in the release of a Dupuytren's contracture where it was felt that there was going to be a significant shortage of skin. **A** The preoperative markings are planned out. **B** The proximally based axial flag flap is being elevated from the proximal phalangeal area of the adjacent finger. It is then transferred through the opened web space. **C** Its appearance on the volar surface. **D** The flaps in place.

Bone exposed with loss of more than half of the nailbed

In this situation, attempts at nail preservation are often ill-advised. The nailbed should be ablated and the bone shortened to allow the remaining local skin to cover the stump. The bone should only be shortened to the insertion of the flexor digitorum profundus (FDP) and extensor tendons. If further shortening is deemed essential to obtain cover, the base of the distal phalanx, the DIP joint and the head of the middle phalanx should all be excised, so that on making a fist the stump is recessed behind the other bones. This prevents its easy exposure to trauma, which would occur if the stump protruded beyond the joint line. The nailbed ablation can be combined with cross-finger or other flaps to preserve the base of the distal phalanx with its attached flexor and extensor tendons if the retention of maximal power grip is vital.

Single middle-segment skin loss

Small narrow bands of contracture can often be released and redundant lateral skin transposed to replace skin loss with a Z-plasty technique. Larger transversely orientated areas of skin loss with exposed vital structures can be repaired by a transposition flap from the midaxial line of the digit. Larger defects require a cross-finger flap for closure. A transposition flap orientated obliquely across the dorsum of the digit, and based on one or other side of the finger, can be elevated to be transposed on to the volar surface of the finger. This flap has limited application because its geometry and short viable flap length make volar transposition difficult.

Single proximal-segment skin loss

Band contractures and small areas of horizontally orientated skin loss can be treated as for similar middle-segment defects. Additional techniques available in the proximal segment are the flag flap, the dorsal rotation flap and the seagull flap.

The arterialized flag flap modified from the middle-segment flag flap of Iselin (1973) is made more reliable by incorporating the dorsal metacarpal artery and draining veins in its flagpole pedicle (Fig. 3.4). The arteries lie on the radial side of the index and middle fingers, allowing elevation of the skin of the dorsal proximal segment from the PIP joint crease, based on the flagpole pedicle. This pedicle must be one-third the width of the flap. The flap is elevated between the subcutaneous fat and the paratenon, and can be transposed through the interdigital cleft to replace the volar proximal-segment skin, interphalangeal web or distal palmar skin.

The dorsal rotation flap is useful for resurfacing the proximal volar segment after the release of severe Dupuytren's contracture (Fig. 3.5). The flap is a true rotation flap, based on the midaxial line of the digit and incorporating the proximal oblique branch of the volar digital artery. It is marked distally at the PIP joint extension crease and along the contralateral midaxial line. A back cut at the MP joint extension crease facilitates transposition.

The seagull flap is useful for syndactyly release, as it simultaneously deepens the web space and releases volar digital contractures at the MP joint level on two adjacent digits (Smith & Harrison 1982; Fig. 3.6). This flap is like two abutting flag flaps on a common flagpole, with two wings or flags draping over the dorsal curvature of the proximal dorsal segment of the digits. The width of the common flagpole or pedicle of the flap should be one-third of the total width of the flap. The flaps are elevated above the paratenon and the cleft adhesions released to abduct the digits fully. The flap is then passed into the web space and the wings are sutured into the volar digital skin defect. This flap avoids a transverse scar across the web margin, hence minimizing web creep.

Multiple-segment volar digital skin loss

Multisegment cross-finger flaps are possible for resurface multisegment volar skin loss on the adjacent digit. This is mentioned only to be deprecated as a technique, because it necessitates the removal of the skin over the dorsum of the PIP joint of the donor digit. Replacement of the skin by full-thickness skin graft is inadequate to restore the full range of movement to the PIP joint, and so this technique effectively sacrifices one finger in an attempt to reconstruct another. Multi-segment skin loss is better treated by distant flap reconstruction.

First-web skin loss

Maintenance of the first web is vital to allow full thumb abduction and maximum hand span. Skin loss can be 'linear' or 'sheet'. Linear constriction bands can be released by Z-plasty techniques, which are useful for lengthening web contracture and deepening a shallow interdigital cleft to create a widened thumb–index interval for the phalangization of a short thumb (Fig. 3.7).

The simplest is the standard two-flap Z-plasty (Fig. 3.7). Under regional anaesthesia and tourniquet control, the distal web ridge is marked from 1 cm proximal to the confluence of the proximal palmar and thenar palmar creases, to the proximal thumb crease. Two lines of equal length are mapped at 60° to the ends of the longitudinal axis line. The distal limb is marked on the dorsal web skin and the proximal limb on the volar skin. The flaps are elevated and the underlying fibrous bands or joint adhesions released, to fully mobilize the first metacarpal. The flaps are then transposed and sutured. A modification of this technique has been described (Woolf & Broadbent 1972; Fig. 3.7D) which allows greater lengthening of the central limb without requiring as much unscarred dorsal or volar web skin adjacent to the contraction band. The central limb is planned as for the two-flap Z-plasty. The dorsal distal and proximal volar limbs are then planned, each equal in length to the central limb and at an angle of 90–120° instead of the 60° in the two-flap Z-plasty. These distal and proximal angles are then each bisected with another limb of equal length to the central member, thus creating four triangular flaps. These are all elevated on their bases and interdigitated such that the central two flaps transpose to the opposite ends of the Z-plasty and the two end flaps abut in the centre of the resulting zigzag suture line.

A five-flap technique has also been described, interposing a V-Y advancement between two adjacent standard two-flap Z-plasties. This gives even greater lengthening of the central member,

without the need for any additional lateral laxity.

Sheet contractures of the first web require more radical solutions to introduce sufficient tissue bulk to maintain adequate release. Small areas of skin deficit can be replaced by proximally based flaps on the dorsum of the hand, overlying the second and third metacarpal heads and extending if necessary along the proximal phalanx of the index. This flap can be elevated above the paratenon and transposed into the released web, and the secondary defect covered by a split-skin graft.

Larger skin requirements can be met by a distally based reversed radial forearm island flap (see Chapter 4), augmented if necessary by a draining subcutaneous vein coapted by microvascular techniques to the cephalic vein in the anatomical snuffbox. Other alternatives are either distant-pedicle two-stage flaps, or microsurgical free flap transfer. This last alternative is the most appropriate, as it combines the ability to elevate the limb and to institute movement in the immediate postoperative period with the importation of large volumes of tissue to allow full web release (Fig. 3.8).

Thumb

Thumbtip amputations can be dealt with in accordance with the principles described for skin loss in the fingertips, except that bone shortening to achieve skin closure is not an option. Length must be preserved, and if at all possible, the skin flap should be sensate. These difficult prerequisites makes a standard cross-finger flap from the dorsal proximal segment of the index a less attractive option than in fingertip injuries. A modification of this technique, described by Foucher & Braun (1979), raises the dorsal proximal segment skin as a neurovascular island, based on the dorsal metacarpal artery and the radial nerve. Under regional anaesthesia and tourniquet exsanguination, the first dorsal metacarpal artery is exposed at its origin through an S-shaped incision in the first interosseous space. The aponeurosis and perivascular fat are raised, with two superficial draining veins and branches of the radial nerve. The radial edge of the skin paddle over the proximal segment is raised next, to minimize the risk of

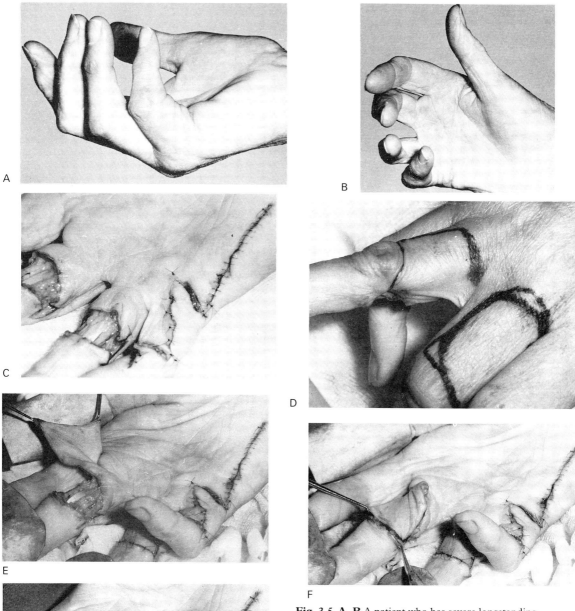

Fig. 3.5 A, B A patient who has severe longstanding Dupuytren's contracture with pronounced flexion deformities affecting both MP and PIP joints. **C** Correction has been achieved with transverse release of the Dupuytren's tissue in the middle and ring fingers, and a longitudinal release and Z-plasties in the little finger. **D** The plan of the dorsal rotation flap. Note that there is a substantial back cut. This flap is based on the oblique proximal branch of the volar digital artery. **E** The flap has been applied to the ring finger and the middle finger flap is being rotated through the second web space. **F** The flap being placed onto the volar surface of the digit. Note the proximal dog-ear. **G** The flap has been sutured in position, full extension of all digits having been achieved. **H, I** The final result with full active extension and flexion.

LOCAL SKIN FLAPS IN THE HAND

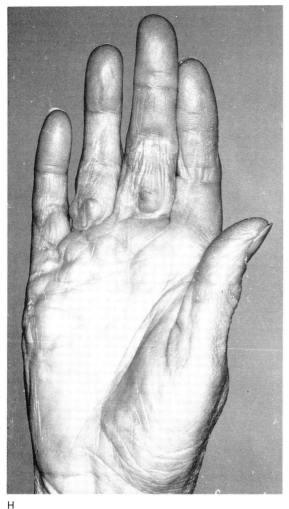

H

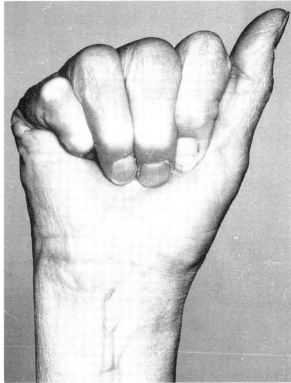

I

Fig. 3.5 Cont'd.

damaging the feeding artery. The rest of the flap is raised superficial to the paratenon. This flap can be transposed to cover defects on the dorsal and ulnar surfaces of the thumb almost to the tip. The problem with this flap is cortical reorientation of sensation.

The radial nerve can be divided and coapted to the stump of the ulnar digital nerve of the thumb, but this does not restore sufficient two-point discrimination to make it preferable to leaving the radial nerve intact. An alternative neurovascular island flap, suitable for skin replacement on the volar surface of the thumbtip, is based on the ulnar neurovascular bundle of the middle finger (Fig. 3.9). This is the preferred site, as it has the longest possible pedicle. Again under regional an-

aesthesia and limb exsanguination, a pattern of the thumb defect is taken and marked onto the ulnar border of the distal segment of the middle finger. An ulnar zigzag incision the length of the digit is made, and the skin flaps are raised to expose the neurovascular pedicle and its surrounding fat. An incision is made in the distal palmar crease and the anatomy of the digital arteries and palmar arch are checked to ensure that isolating the ulnar digital artery of the middle finger does not render either middle or ring fingers ischaemic. If the anatomy proves normal, the flap is incised and the skin of the pulp undermined to include more subcutaneous tissue than skin, to facilitate closure of the secondary defect in the pulp. The flap is then raised from the periosteum of the

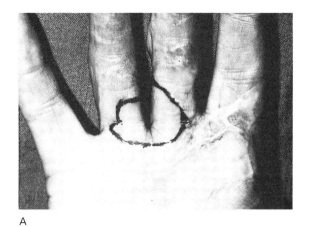

A

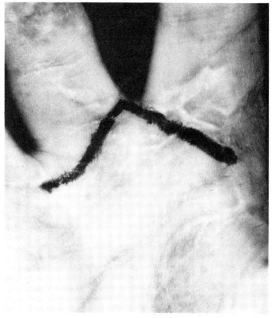

B

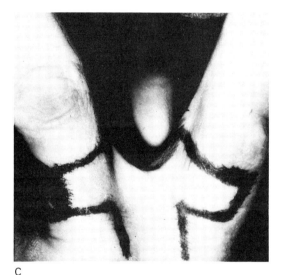

C

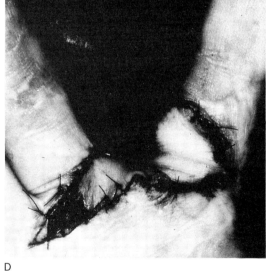

D

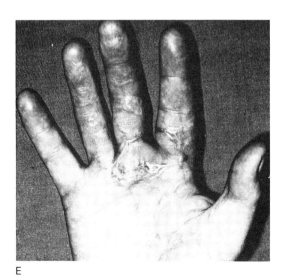

E

Fig. 3.6 The seagull flap for proximal syndactyly. **A** A preoperative photograph shows the second web space which requires release. The third web space is outlined and has been the previous site of a butterfly flap. A good result was obtained. **B** The preoperative markings on the palmar surface of the hand. **C** The preoperative markings on the dorsal surface of the hand. **D** The flap in its new situation. **E** The result some 4 weeks later, with the creation of a good second web space.

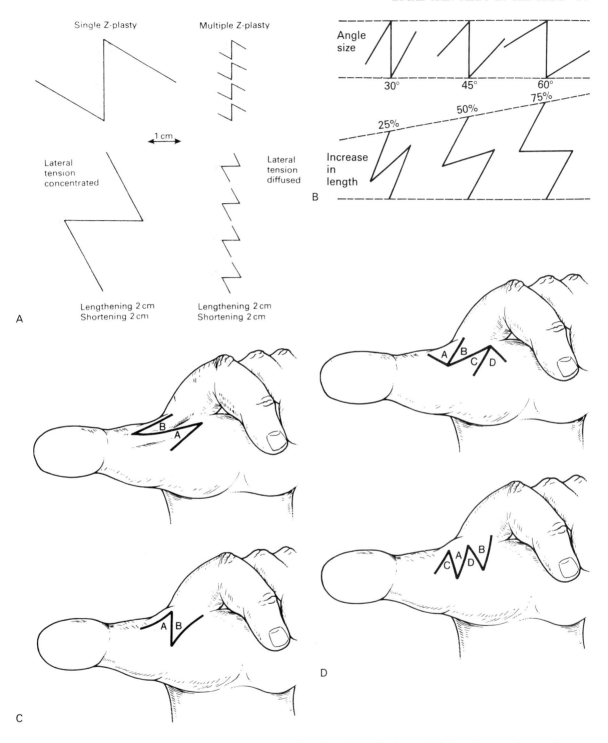

Fig. 3.7 A The principles of a single 60° Z-plasty. Note the effect of a multiple Z-plasty, which gives the same degree of lengthening without the requirement of lax tissues on either side. **B** The effect of altering the angle size on the increase in length of the Z-plasty. It should be noted, however, that in most first-web space releases, Z-plasties are undertaken either at 90° or 120° angles. **C** The effect of a two-flap Z-plasty with a 90° angle on the first web space. **D** A four-flap Z-plasty with four 60° Z-plasties undertaken and positioned as indicated in the lower figure.

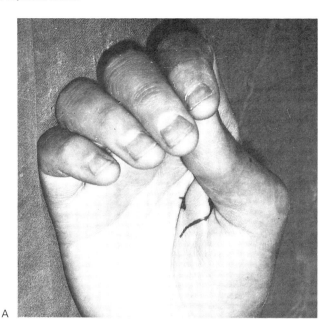

A

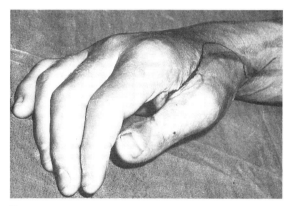

B

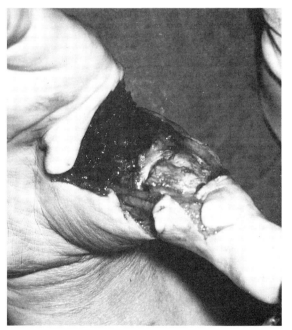

C

Fig. 3.8 A This man sustained a scratch on the dorsum of his first web space which led to a streptococcal infection producing loss of consciousness within 24 hours. He was admitted to hospital unconscious and almost moribund; he was resuscitated, but eventually produced an abscess in the first web space which led to scarring and contracture. He presented with an adducted thumb as shown in the illustration. **B** This shows the dorsal view and the planned release leading up towards the radial artery. A free flap reconstruction was contemplated. **C** The completed release, following skin release, release of the muscle fascia and release of the carpometacarpal joint in order to produce good abduction. **D** A dorsalis pedis flap in position. Note the fact that the flap goes well to the midaxial line of the thumb on the radial side. **E** The dorsal view of the first web space with the dorsalis pedis flap in position.

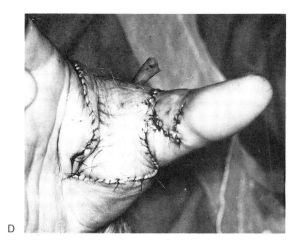

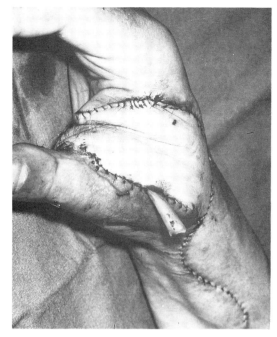

Fig. 3.8 Cont'd.

distal phalanx and the pedicle dissected free, preserving a cuff of surrounding fat to minimize spasm and retain some draining veins. At the bifurcation of the common digital artery in the palm, the radial digital artery to the ring finger is divided, and frequently the division of the common digital nerve has to be split proximally to mobilize the pedicle adequately and allow transposition. A wide subcutaneous tunnel is then developed from the palm along the volar surface of the thumb to the defect on the thumb pulp. The flap is then passed through the tunnel, taking care to avoid twisting the pedicle. The donor site can often be closed directly, or is repaired with a split-skin graft. Again, lack of cortical reorientation is the major disadvantage with this technique, especially in those over 40 years of age. However, digital nerve division and coaptation to the thumb digital nerve, or free pulp transfer both fail to restore sensation as completely as the pedicled neurovascular island flap.

Palm

Small distal palmar defects are suitable for flaps from the dorsal proximal phalangeal segment, such as the flag flap or the seagull flap. More proximal transverse skin loss with intact distal palmar skin can be dealt with by the McCash open palm technique, or if a finger is too severely injured or involved with Dupuytren's contracture to be restored to useful function, it can be sacrificed and filleted of its skeleton and tendons, leaving the skin to be transposed into the palm. More proximal small areas of skin loss can be dealt with by local rotation or advancements flaps. These techniques are of limited application because of the multiple septae binding the palmar skin, the lack of redundancy of the palmar skin and because of its limited intrinsic elasticity. Larger areas of skin loss necessitate distant pedicled or free flap transfer, as resistance to contracture formation, sensory return and durability are all highly desirable qualities in a palmar reconstruction. These three qualities are more likely to be obtained by a vascularized flap transfer than by split-skin grafting, although Wolfe grafts have a place.

DORSAL SKIN

Although there is an apparent excess of dorsal skin as compared with the volar surface of the hand and digits, the dorsal skin has little transverse

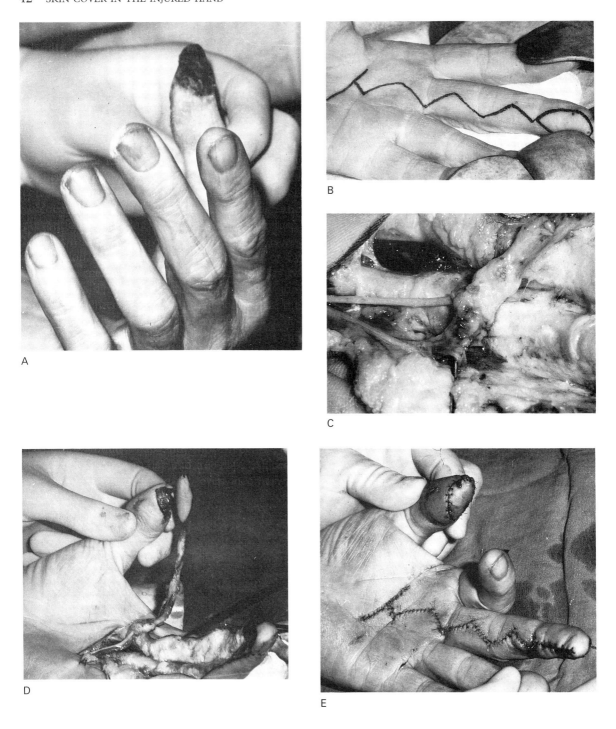

Fig. 3.9 The neurovascular island flap. **A** A necrotic thumbtip following a crush injury to the finger. **B** The plan of a neurovascular island flap from the ulnar side of the long finger. **C** The preliminary check that is always made to ensure that there is a blood supply to the ulnar side of the ring finger, so that when the radial vessel is divided to allow mobilization of the neurovascular island flap, one is sure that the vascularity of the ring finger is intact. **D** The neurovascular island flap. Note how easily it reaches the tip of the thumb. **E** The neurovascular island flap in place. The donor defect has been closed directly. **F** The eventual result of the neurovascular island flap.

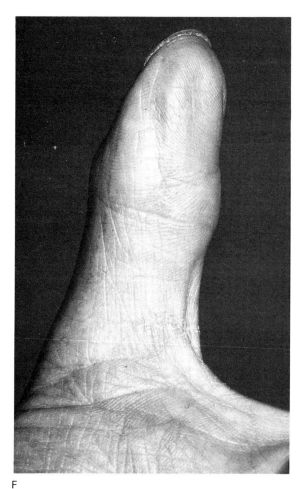

F

Fig. 3.9 Cont'd.

distensibility and its elasticity in the longitudinal axis is needed to allow the full range of joint flexion. The dorsum is the surface most exposed to trauma because the functional position of the hand for most activities requires joint flexion. In this position the skin over the joints is more vulnerable to injury and skin loss. Areas of skin loss can be single or multiple; if single, they can be orientated transversely, obliquely or longitudinally in relationship to the long axis of the finger.

A transverse defect, if small, can be treated by taking a conventional transposition flap from the adjacent intact dorsal skin and replacing the skin in the secondary defect with a skin graft. A greater arc of rotation of the transposition flap can be obtained by releasing Cleland's ligaments, which bind the dorsal skin to the underlying phalanx at the midlateral line just dorsal to the neurovascular bundle. These transposition flaps must have a wide base, as the blood supply from the dorsal skin arises from the digital arteries and runs dorsally and obliquely distally. Therefore narrow-based transverse flaps would have no intact artery running the length of the long axis of the flap. The full width of the cosmetic unit or segment would be the safest design for these transposition flaps. Another limitation of their design is that, on transposition, the line of greatest tension from the pivot point to the point of maximum movement would come to lie across the dorsum of the joint. Therefore on healing there is a dorsal linear line of tension restricting joint flexion and thus limiting early mobilization.

An alternative flap for small transverse defects on the dorsum of the digit, with intact lateral digital skin, is that described by Leuders and Shapiro (1971). These flaps are based proximally on the lateral surface of the PIP joint and outlined on this intact lateral skin to the level of the DIP joint. These flaps can be raised by a length-to-breadth ratio of 3:1, and can then be transposed across the dorsum of the PIP joint. The secondary defect is covered by a full-thickness skin graft.

Obliquely orientated defects can be repaired by using a sliding transposition flap (Smith 1982; Fig. 3.10). This is best suited to elliptical defects. The flap is designed to lie on the side of the defect with the most redundant skin. A line is drawn extending in a projection of the curve of the side of the defect furthest from the proposed flap; this line is made the same length as the defect – this is the distal margin of the flap. The second line is then drawn, initially parallel to the ipsilateral curve of the defect, to a point opposite the maximal width of the defect. Thereafter the margin of the flap diverges from the margin of the defect to increase the width of the base of the flap. The proximal limit of this line is opposite the proximal extent of the skin defect. The flap is then raised superficial to the paratenon and is folded back on itself, so that the point of the flap at the distal end of the defect is transposed back to the proximal end of the defect and the distal end of the flap covers the distal end of the skin defect. Where the flap folds on itself there is a prominent dog-ear. The secondary defect is covered with a full-

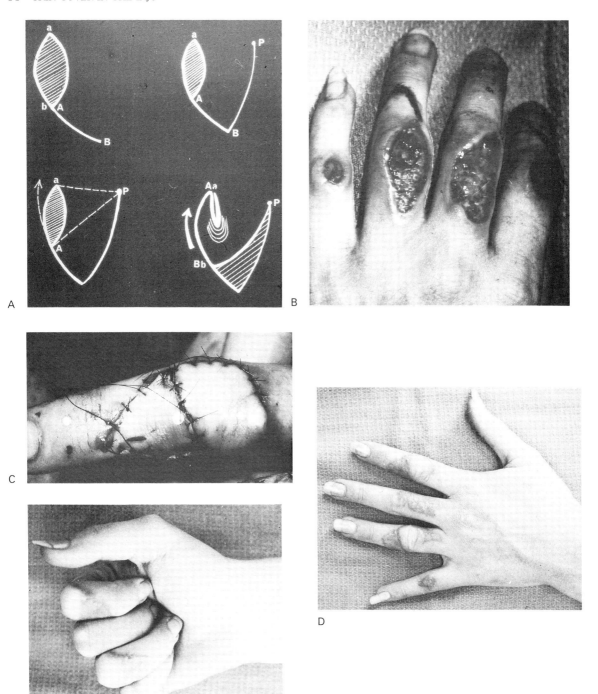

Fig. 3.10 The sliding transposition flap. **A** The sequence of planning the flap. A line is projected to the length of one side of the defect, i.e. AB = ab. Then another line is projected commencing parallel to the ipsilateral side of the defect and running towards P. It can be seen that PA exceeds Pa, so that when the flap is transposed a dog-ear results, and the tension across the flap in its transposed state is less than the tension in its original situation. **B** This patient is suitable for a sliding transposition flap. The index and middle fingers have bony exposure and need sliding transposition flaps, whereas the ring and little fingers simply require skin grafts. **C** The sliding transposition flap in position, with the secondary defect grafted. **D** The result at 4 weeks, with full extension of the digits. **E** The result at 4 weeks with full flexion.

thickness skin graft. The advantages of this flap are firstly that the obliquity of its design is better orientated to coincide with the obliquely running arterial supply to the dorsal digital skin, giving the flap a more reliable vascular basis, and secondly, that there is less tension along the pivot line of the flap after transposition. Indeed, careful design can often position the dog-ear over the PIP joint, thus providing a useful skin redundancy in an area where skin laxity helps early joint mobilization. With time the dog-ear settles, but the skin redundancy remains a functional advantage.

Small longitudinal areas of skin loss can often be dealt with by raising the skin adjacent to the defect as a longitudinal bipedicle flap, and advancing it transversely across the finger to cover the defect. This has limited application, as advancement around the convex surface is always less than expected.

Large defects can be dealt with by cross-finger flaps, either a flag flap from the same segment of an adjacent digit or alternatively a reverse-dermis flap (see Chapter 5). This latter flap, described by Pakiam (1978), is raised as a standard transverse cross-finger flap, except that the segment is deepithelialized prior to raising the flap. The flap is designed so that its base is adjacent to the digit with the area of skin loss, and it is transposed by turning it over, so that the deepithelialized dermis is placed on the exposed structures and the subcutaneous fat of the deep surface of the flap is left uppermost and exposed, thus requiring a skin graft to cover both flap and secondary defect. This technique can lead to the problems of two-stage immobilization and joint stiffness common to all cross-finger techniques, but it also has some unique problems intrinsic to its design. It may be a disadvantage to place dermis directly over exposed tendon, joint or bone, and there may be complications related to the burying of dermal elements, mainly inclusion cysts and buried hair growth.

Multiple areas of skin loss, or large areas, necessitate distant flap transfer.

Dorsum of hand

Small areas of skin loss on the dorsum of the hand can be filled by utilizing adjacent skin laxity, with local transposition or rotation flap techniques. Larger areas necessitate either the reversed radial forearm fasciocutaneous flap, or distant flap transfer, either using staged pedicle techniques or free tissue transfer (see Chapters 5, and 7–11).

CONCLUSIONS

The replacement of highly specialized skin of the hand by 'like' skin is a reconstructive ideal. However, this is often difficult because there is little redundant skin in the hand and normal hand function necessitates a degree of skin laxity to allow full range of movement. Various techniques have been outlined in the different anatomical areas of the hand to try and achieve this reconstructive ideal. The selection of the most appropriate technique for a given patient with a unique problem is dependent on the surgeon's assessment of the patient and his injury.

REFERENCES

Atasoy E, Ioakimidis E, Kasdan M L et al 1970
   Reconstruction of the amputated finger tip with a triangular volar flap. Journal of Bone and Joint Surgery 52A: 921
Evans D M, Martin D L 1988 Step-advancement island flap for finger tip reconstruction. British Journal of Plastic Surgery 41: 105
Foucher G, Braun J B 1979 A new island flap transfer from the dorsum of the index to the thumb. Plastic and Reconstructive Surgery 63: 344
Iselin F 1973 The flag flap. Plastic and Reconstructive Surgery 52: 374
Leuders H W, Shapiro R L 1971 Rotation finger flaps in reconstruction of burned hands. Plastic and Reconstructive Surgery 47: 176
Pakiam A I 1978 The reverse dermis flap. British Journal of Plastic Surgery 31: 131
Smith P J 1982 A sliding flap to cover dorsal skin defects over the proximal interphalangeal joint. Hand 14: 271
Smith P J, Harrison S H 1982 The 'seagull' flap for syndactyly. British Journal of Plastic Surgery 35: 390
Tranquilli-Leali E 1935 Reconstruzione dell'apice delle falangi ungueali mediante autoplastica volare peduncolata per scorrimento. Infost. Traum. Lavoro l: 186
Venkataswami R, Subramanian N 1980 Oblique triangular flap: a new method of repair for oblique amputations of the fingertip and thumb. Plastic and Reconstructive Surgery 66: 296
Woolf R M, Broadbent T R 1972 The four-flap Z-plasty. Plastic and Reconstructive Surgery 49: 48

The radial forearm flap in surgery of the hand

The radial forearm flap is a fasciocutaneous flap based on the radial artery. It was first described in China in 1978, and details were published in 1981 (Yang et al 1981, Song et al 1982). The senior author has used it since 1980, having seen it in China during the first French microsurgery mission to that country, and has modified the flap utilizing it as a composite flap containing bone, muscle or tendon (Foucher 1982, Foucher et al 1984a, b, 1987). It can also be used with only the fascia (Yang et al 1981, Schoofs et al 1983), and transferred either as a free or an island flap. This flap raises several questions of haemodynamics. As a free flap it has high perfusion pressure inflow. Used as an island flap, it receives retrograde perfusion through the radial artery, whose anastomosis with the ulnar artery is constant, but the venous return by the venae comitantes might be worrying because of a reverse flow and because of the presence of valves.

ANATOMICAL BASIS

The radial artery, whose mean diameter is 1.9 mm with a range of 1.6–2.6 mm, (Braun 1977), arises most often in the centre of the antecubital fossa and descends deep to the brachioradialis before becoming more superficial in the distal third of the forearm. It then spirals around the wrist, crossing the anatomical snuff box before passing into the space between the first and second metacarpals. Not only can its origin vary (high origin in 2% of cases) but it can also be very slender (1.5%) and in this case it is associated with a larger superficial dorsal forearm artery

(Braun 1984). The authors have encountered this type of distribution in one case, but it did not prevent the successful raising of an island flap. Other variations have been mentioned (Yang et al 1981, Braun 1977, Timmons et al 1986, Small & Millar 1985, Fatah & Davies 1984).

There is a large number of side branches 1–2 cm apart in the distal half of the forearm (from 9 to 17 in all) (Timmons 1986) the proximal ones being less numerous but usually larger. Longitudinal connections have been demonstrated by several authors (Manchot 1983, Timmons 1986). Two arteries appear to be more constant: one destined to supply the distal forearm skin leaves the arterial trunk 7 cm above the radial styloid; the other, slimmer, one leaves at 2–5 cm above the radial styloid and plunges into the pronator quadratus, ending in the radial epiphysis. This branch is used in the composite osteocutaneous flap; the vascularization of the distal radius was confirmed by Cormack et al (1986).

In the distal part it is important to know the artery's connections and how it branches, because the reverse flow of an island flap depends on these features. In the region of the radial pulse there is a superficial palmar branch which is constant, but less commonly anastomoses with the ulnar artery (7 out of 30 according to Braun, 1977). This calls into question the notion of a constant superficial arcade. More distally, Gelberman et al (1983) have given an excellent description of the three dorsal and palmar arcades of the wrist, the two constant ones being the dorsal intercarpal and the palmar radiocarpal. They have also shown that the radial artery is not indispensable for the blood supply of the bones of the carpus. Distally the radial artery is continuous with the ulnar artery in two-thirds of the population; however, even if there is no direct connection, anastomotic branches are constant.

A study of the arterial flows performed in situ by Khashaba and MacGregor (1986) did not show any significant difference between antegrade flow (4.65 + 1.2 ml/min) and retrograde flow (4.8 + 1.13 ml/min). The net flow seems to vary according to temperature and the surface area of the flap.

CUTANEOUS TERRITORY

Clinical and cadaveric injection studies (Foucher 1982) showed that a large part of the skin of the forearm can be based solely on the radial artery. Yang et al (1981) have found that in clinical situations almost the whole of the skin of the forearm, and even part of the inferior quarter of the anterior skin of the arm, can be harvested. When taking a more conventionally sized flap, the authors usually align it so that one-third of the surface area is radial and two-thirds are ulnar to the vascular axis.

VENOUS DRAINAGE

Venous drainage is via two systems, superficial and deep, with many anastomoses. For free flaps we use the superficial vein known as the cephalic, which lies on the radial border of the flap and which must not be separated from the skin. This vein has many tiny anastomotic connections with other superficial branches and with the deep system. Timmons (1986) noted in 7 out of 11 forearms a large communicating vein between the superficial and deep network, 6–7.5 cm from the radial styloid. When taking the flap as an island, the cephalic vein is often left in situ, the venous drainage being left to venae comitantes which run alongside the artery. Their dissection needs care, and haemostasis of their afferent branches must be performed at a distance from the trunk when using bipolar coagulation. Oedema of the island flap is frequently noted in the first 72 hours, but this is not found in free flaps with a venous repair

in the normal direction of venous flow. It has been well shown that the deep veins have valves, to an even greater extent than the superficial venous system (Timmons 1986). The theory proposed by Lin et al (1984) was that these valves were by-passed by collateral flow, but this was not clearly demonstrated in their study. On the other hand, Emerson, quoted by Timmons (1986), has shown retrograde filling of both venae comitantes after injecting one, but eventual obstruction by valves in both veins. Timmons confirmed that at some stage in distally based island flaps the blood has to flow through valves. This is possible if three conditions are all fulfilled: denervation, blood in the vein proximal and distal to the valve, and higher venous blood pressure proximal to the valve than distal to it. Lastly it is interesting to note the haemodynamic study of Khashaba and McGregor (1986), which did not show any significant difference between the efficiency of the two venous systems.

SENSORY INNERVATION

The sensory acuity of the flap territory is poor when assessed by two-point discrimination. The authors found better discrimination in the distal forearm and in a transverse direction. It varies from 30.7 mm proximally to 16.8 mm at around the level of the radial pulse. Two-point discrimination of the forearm varies in the same areas from 36.5 mm (longitudinal axis) to 18.5 mm (transverse direction) (Braun 1984, Braun et al 1985).

Depending on the site and size of the flap, up to three nerves can usually be included in the flap: on the radial side, the sensory branch of the radial nerve and the lateral cutaneous nerve of the forearm, and anteriorly the medial cutaneous nerve of the forearm. The authors have frequently found an anastomosis between the radial nerve and the lateral cutaneous nerve of the forearm (60%) between 4 and 8 cm from the radial styloid. The lateral cutaneous nerve of the forearm frequently included in the authors' flap is easily found on the lateral border of the biceps tendon. It then runs along the accessory cephalic vein and often ends in two branches. Its diameter and its fascicular structure are very close to that of a digital nerve, with 26.2% as opposed to 26.7% of its cross-sectional area occupied by fascicles. The authors have never used the radial nerve, which is carefully dissected and left undisturbed.

SURGICAL TECHNIQUES

Preoperative investigations

In addition to routine investigations, the circulation in the hand without input from the radial artery should be assessed. In elective cases the authors do not perform either preoperative arteriography or Doppler studies (Jones & O'Brien 1985): Allen's test (Allen 1929) is sufficient, provided it is timed properly as Gelberman and Blasinghame (1981) proposed. The filling time after release of the radial or ulnar artery is less than 3 seconds. In emergency cases the test can be carried out after exsanguination of the arm and inflation of the tourniquet. Clamping of the radial artery and tourniquet release enables the circulation in the hand to be checked.

The operation

The majority of the authors' patients requiring this flap are treated as day cases, except those with free flaps who are hospitalized for 5 days. We have never noted a vascular complication to occur after this time. The operation is usually performed with the patient supine, with an axillary regional anaesthetic block and a tourniquet on the upper arm. The design of the flap is variable, depending on the size required and the length of the vascular pedicle. Whether it is being designed high or low on the forearm, it is still designed one-third radial, two-thirds ulnar with respect to the axis of the radial artery. It is preferable to take the forearm fascia with the flap when the flap is being taken from a proximal site (to provide a longer pedicle) or when the flap is of a large size. Including the fascia safeguards the longitudinal connections on the superficial aspects of the fascia, which permits safe enlargement of the area of the flap.

For a distally based island flap the first stage is to locate the radial vessels at the proximal border of the flap. At this level the pedicle is tied, the veins and arteries being tied separately, and the

artery is henceforth kept as one with the skin and subcutaneous tissue of the flap. The skin is thereafter perpendicularly incised straight through fat, right down to and including the fascia. This should also be raised in one block with the skin. The flap is then raised from the underlying muscle from the ulnar border as far as the lateral border of the flexor digitorum superficialis, and from the radial border as far as the anterior aspect of the

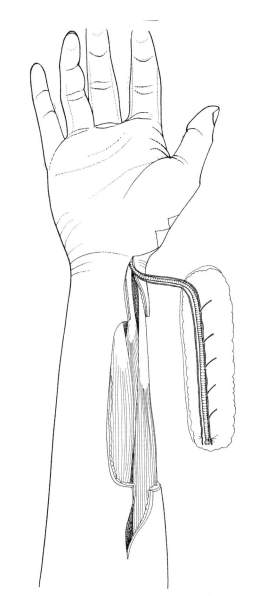

Fig. 4.1 A distally based radial forearm island flap raised, with dissection of the vascular pedicle as far as the wrist crease.

brachioradialis. The branches of the lateral cutaneous nerve, close to the axis of the vascular pedicle, are identified and dissected as necessary. Care must be taken in the distal third of the forearm to identify and leave in situ the superficial branch of the radial nerve, which emerges at the posterior border of the tendon of the brachioradialis. The flap is now attached only by its septum, which contains the supplying vessels. The dissection then proceeds from proximal to distal, lifting the flap progressively and performing haemostasis on the numerous muscular branches (Fig. 4.1). The distal part of the pedicle is freed until the radial artery passes beneath the tendon of abductor pollicis longus (Fig. 4.2). The dissection can stop there, keeping the thenar muscular branch of the radial artery, which must not be kinked when the flap is turned distally. Because of the risk of compression the authors have only rarely used a palmar tunnel. If the pedicle needs to be longer the dissection of the radial artery can be continued beneath the tendon of the long abductor, short extensor and long extensor of the thumb, so that the flap and artery can be disentangled from these superficial tendons by passing

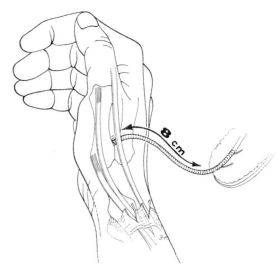

Fig. 4.3 Further dissection of the pedicle and passage of the flap beneath the tendons to the thumb gives an additional 5 cm of pedicle length, with a more distal pivoting point and much greater range.

the flap through the space (Fig. 4.3). This is tedious and exacting, due to the fact that there are many side branches going to the wrist bones. The studies of Gelberman et al (1983) have shown, however, that division of these carpal branches does not have any adverse effects on the vascularization of the carpus because of the richness of the anastomotic arcades. It is thus possible to dissect the artery and two veins until they disappear into the first metacarpal interspace. This uncrossing manoeuvre elongates the pedicle by 8 cm. Such a distal dissection is contraindicated in cases when the first commissure is damaged. Venous drainage will then be required through more proximal veins associated with the carpal arteries.

The dissection of a free radial forearm flap is also simple, the freeing of the pedicle being more limited. Care is needed not to separate the cephalic vein from the radial border of the flap. It is also important to prepare the correct length of pedicle, depending on the type of reconstruction. An orthograde circulation is preferable in both the arterial and the venous systems. For example, when the flap is used on the back of the hand, the arterial anastomosis can be made end-to-end via a venous bridge graft sutured proximally to the cut end of the radial artery. For the venous

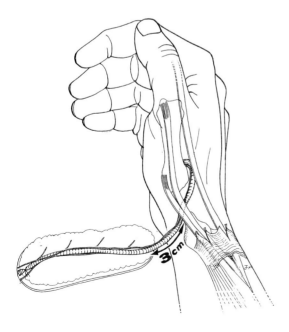

Fig. 4.2 Dissection of the pedicle as far as the tendon of abductor pollicis longus, giving limited range to the flap.

anastomosis it is preferable to suture the proximal stump of the cephalic vein end-to-end with a vein on the back of the forearm. Once the flap has been tacked into position, the authors do not hesitate to perform Z-plasties immediately in view of the excellent vascularization of these flaps. We have also made perforations in order to pass fingers 'through' the flap. In this case care is needed to avoid damaging the pedicle. The donor site can be treated in various ways. With narrow flaps it is sometimes possible to close the donor site by direct suture. In emergency cases one can delay the graft, even if it can be taken under local anaesthetic. The edges of the defect are brought closer to each other by means of thick sutures over a stent, in order to prevent the normal retraction of the edges which would increase the area. Grafts can also be applied immediately. Thin grafts have the advantage that they tend to retract and thus decrease the extent of the scar. In a woman, the use of a tissue expander might be possible as a secondary procedure, followed by excision of the graft.

Variations

Several variations are possible. An island flap can be used in different situations: with a distal pedicle as has been described; with a proximal pedicle, for repair of skin loss in the region of the elbow and of the arm; and, rarely, the flap can be used as a cross-forearm island flap in cases of injury (and repair) of both the main vessels of the hand, mainly if a secondary free transfer (e.g. second toe) is planned. The flap can also be used as a bipedicle flap, which is almost ideal because it does not interrupt the radial circulation. The authors have used it in two indications: one as a skin flap to replace a thick scar after multiple operations and to cover a fascicular nerve graft of the median nerve; also a bipedicled fascial flap has been used to provide increased blood supply in a case of Volkmann's contracture, the flap being wrapped around the median nerve after neurolysis and excision of the surrounding fibrous tissue.

Fascial flap

This can be used with or without a paddle of skin,

the fascial flap greatly exceeding the cutaneous one in size, and large enough to be wrapped as a tube around a nerve, nerve grafts or tendons. It can also bring an ideal sliding sheath or a capillary bed which can improve the vascularity of the structure it surrounds. The fascial flap is also indicated in obese people, where the forearm flap would be too thick. The fascia can be grafted with split- or full-thickness skin. The donor site of the latter can generally be sutured directly.

Composite flaps

The flap can contain vascularized nerve, muscle, tendon or bone, (Fig. 4.4). The authors have attempted to reinnervate the flap in four cases: the lateral antebrachial cutaneous nerve was sutured to a digital or radial nerve, giving two-point discrimination of 9 mm on the radial side of the flap in one case, and protective sensibility only in three cases.

It is also possible to incorporate tendons in the flap to repair, for example, the loss of the extensor apparatus on the back of the hand, ensuring that the tendons are vascularized. It is possible to use the brachioradialis divided into several strips distally for this purpose. Two other tendons can be prepared: the flexor carpi radialis, which can be half stripped (but its dissection and elevation are delicate), and the palmaris longus. A composite cutaneotendinous flap is actually easier to position as a free flap, as opposed to as an island flap.

Lastly, incorporation of a small vascularized bone graft is of particular value, notably in one-stage reconstruction of the thumb. The authors performed their first case in 1980 (Foucher 1982). This technique has also been used by others (Biemer & Stock 1983, Soutar & Tanner 1984). The authors prefer to take the matchstick of bone graft from the distal part of the radius (Fig. 4.1A–F). Its removal is delicate because a fringe of the pronator quadratus must be removed en bloc with the flap, together with the small bone graft. It is advisable to prepare the bone cuts with a drill and then to complete them with an osteotome. Some authors have noted radial fractures (Timmons et al 1986), but this is a complication which the authors have not had in their series due to the small size of the bone grafts and to their donor site being in the widest part of the radius. In the majority of the authors' cases (6 out of 11) of one-stage osteoplastic reconstructions we proceeded at a second stage to a sensory island flap transfer according to Littler (1956).

INDICATIONS

The forearm flap possesses most of the qualities one would wish for in a flap for use in the hand:

- Its elasticity corresponds well to the needs of dorsal skin cover, but less well for those of palmar skin cover, where its thickness and its mobility are sometimes a hindrance in grip.
- Its colour is satisfactory.
- Its ability to be used in cases requiring a large flap is very important. The authors have used it in three cases of near-total hand degloving.

- Its vascular reliability is excellent and the authors have not seen any failure in a series of 53 flaps in 52 patients, of which 47 were island flaps.
- The size of its pedicle facilitates its use as a free flap.
- The flap possesses its own vascular supply, which means that it does not act as a parasite: on the contrary, it brings extra blood supply to the surrounding structures. Its pedicle can also be used to revascularize a finger in the acute situation (two cases) or secondarily to supply a free toe transfer (two cases).
- Skin cover using this flap can be carried out as a one-stage procedure using the same operating field and local anaesthesia, thus facilitating its use in emergency cases (12 cases out of 53) and out-patient surgery.
- It can be used as a compound flap with tendons (Reid and Moss 1983, Foucher et al

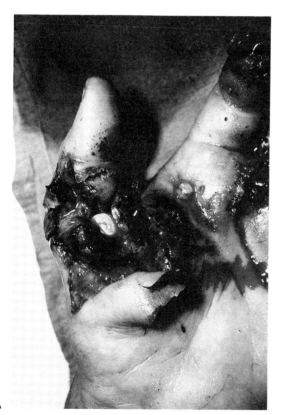 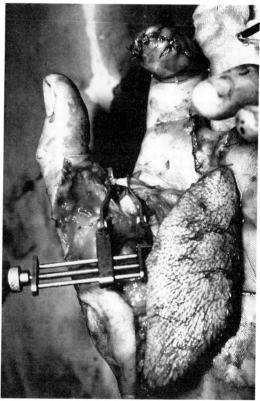

A　　　　　　　　　　　　　　　　　　　　　B

Fig. 4.4　A A severe compound injury of the thumb with loss of skin and bone, and neurovascular disruption.
B Reconstruction using a compound transfer of skin and a piece of bone from the radius as a distally based radial forearm island flap. Sensation is provided by nerve repair to the medial cutaneous nerve of the forearm, and the radial artery has been anastomosed to the ulnar digital artery of the thumb. **C** A diagram of the anatomical rearrangement. **D, E, F** The healed functional result. **G** The donor site.

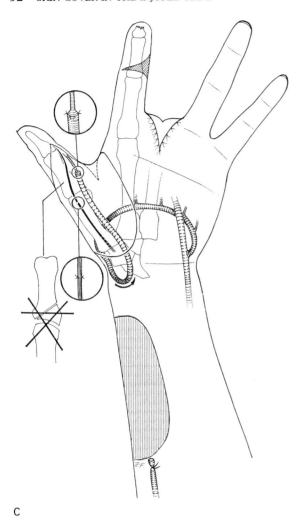

C

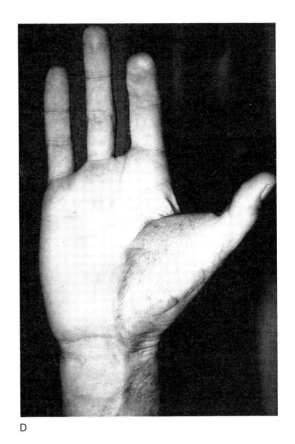

D

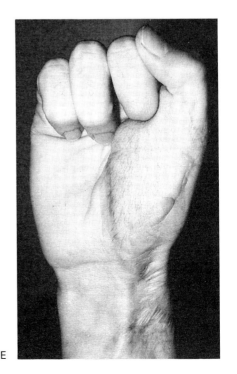

E

Fig. 4.4 Cont'd.

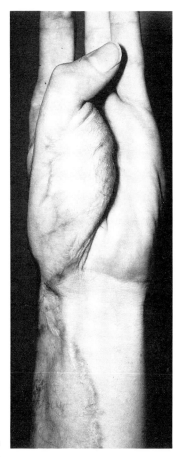

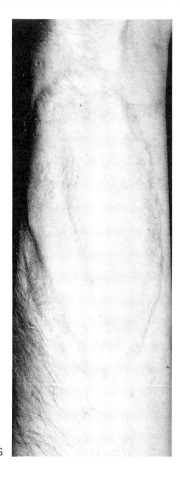

F   G

Fig. 4.4 Cont'd.

1984a) or bone (Foucher 1982, Biemer & Stock 1983).

• Postoperative mobilization and splinting are greatly facilitated by the use of this flap.

• The flap is more comfortable for the patient than distant pedicle flaps such as the groin flap.

These numerous advantages must not, however, make one forget its two principal disadvantages (Boorman et al 1987, Timmons et al 1986):

1. The sacrifice of the radial artery has not led to any ischaemic complication in our series, but this occurrence has been noted in the literature (Jones & O'Brien 1985), and in this case the problem was overcome with a vein graft. It must, however, be remembered that the majority of problems following procedures on the radial artery reported in the literature were in connection with thrombosis or embolization of the artery after

arterial cannulation. Reconstruction of the radial artery is easy in cases when the flap is taken as a free flap, but it is difficult when it is raised as an island flap. The authors have used vein grafts on five occasions, but two have thrombosed; this confirms the findings of Gelberman et al (1982), with 53% thrombosis of arterial repair in the forearm in non-critical situations.

Intolerance to cold was found in 79% of the authors' cases. However, one cannot regard this complication as a direct consequence of obliteration of the radial artery, because an identical incidence was found in a series of major hand injuries treated in eastern France. Cold intolerance was also found in the three cases in which the radial artery was replaced with a vein graft and the graft remained patent. In nine of the authors' old cases this cold intolerance has markedly decreased after 2 years. Lastly, the authors studied four cases by means of dynamic scintigraphy with Fourier analysis, allowing a quantitative approach. No decrease in peripheral perfusion was noted, which supports Gelberman's view (Gelberman et al 1983).

A decrease in the force of the muscles of the forearm (20%) was frequently found by Legre in a series of cases in which the flap was transferred to the head and neck (Legre et al 1986). The use of the flap on the same side as a complex hand injury does not enable one to make an independent estimation of the decrease in strength of the flexor muscles due to removal of the flap alone, but in two cases where the flap was used on the opposite side, a measure of force was taken both before and after the operation and did not show any significant difference on the donor side.

2. Grafting of the donor site may present three difficulties:

1. Difficulty with 'take' of the graft, especially on bare tendon such as the flexor carpi radialis, has occurred in five cases in the authors' series. The following suggestions have been made in the literature:

(a) Fenton and Roberts (1985) have proposed suturing the muscle bellies of flexor pollicis longus to flexor digitorum superficialis in order to avoid the exposure of moving tendons when taking a large flap.

(b) McGregor (1987) has reported good results following the application of grafts with the wrist held in extension for 2 weeks, in order to achieve good adherence to the underlying flexor carpi radialis tendon.

2. Hypersensitivity was noticed in eight cases, although none of them had a definite painful neuroma. (There was no case among this group in which the radial nerve was taken.)

3. Appearance was a problem only once, in a 52-year-old woman, for whom compensation was a feature. The cosmetic result could be criticised in eight other cases, where there was partial necrosis of the graft leading to hypertrophic scar.

There are other problems concerning the donor site, but only in Caucasians. In the Chinese, the forearm region generally has a thin layer of subcu-

taneous fat and the skin surface is not hairy – it is not always the same in western patients! The presence of a thick layer of subcutaneous fat was a problem in six patients, leading in one case to the use of a fascial flap plus graft in order to cover a large loss of substance in the thumb. In five other cases one or more defattings of the flap were necessary. Lastly the hairiness of the flap, sometimes very marked and rather ugly in the palm or on the thumb, compelled six of our patients to shave the area frequently.

Bearing in mind these advantages and disadvantages, the indications for the radial forearm flap in surgery of the hand have become clearer. The authors have used a total of 53 flaps in patients aged from 9 to 84 years, with a mean age of 34.9 years. The indications were to provide skin cover on the dorsum of the hand including the fingers (26.4%), on the palmar surface only (20.7%), on both the dorsal and palmar surface (5.6%), and in the first web (5.6%). The flap is least satisfactory in the palm due to its bulk and mobility. It shares these inconvenient features with all remote flaps, except the 'flap graft', entirely defatted according to Colson and Janvier (1966), which behaves more like a graft and adheres to the subjacent tissue.

In 34% of the authors' cases the flap was utilized for reconstruction of the thumb. This is a major indication, as it allows a one-stage reconstruction. The vascularized bone graft avoids the resorption frequently seen with non-vascularized bone grafts in classic osteoplastic reconstruction. The authors have observed one case of a true fracture of this bony fragment following a fall onto the thumb. The fracture healed in 3 weeks with a slightly hypertrophic callus. This osteoplastic reconstruction with a composite forearm flap finds its place among techniques available for thumb reconstruction, essentially in subjects aged more than 40 years presenting with an amputation at the level of the metacarpophalangeal joint, and in whom there is no other finger stump which can be pollicized. The elongation obtained is greater than that obtained by using the technique of Matev (1970). When choosing the technique of reconstruction, careful assessment of the range of flexion in the opposing finger is mandatory – the stiffer the finger, the longer the thumb has to be.

The indications for the radial forearm flap need to be considered first in relation to other forearm flaps, then to the groin flap, and lastly in relation to free flaps.

Three skin flaps are comparable to the radial flap: the forearm flap based on the ulnar artery, the flap of Becker centred on an arterial branch of the ulnar artery (Becker, personal communication) and the flap of Zancolli and Angrigiani (1986) and Masquelet and Penteado (1987) based retrogradely on the posterior interosseous vessels. Muscle flaps (resurfaced with a graft) such as the pronator quadratus flap described by Dellon and MacKinnon (1984) have specifically been excluded from our discussion.

The ulnar forearm flap (Lovie et al 1984) has the major theoretical inconvenience of sacrificing the dominant vascular supply to the hand. It does, however, have the advantage of being a less hairy donor site, which is easier to hide. The authors' reserve this flap for amputations of the four long fingers, keeping the radial artery intact for the vascularization of the thumb.

The flap of Becker is based on an artery which supplies skin, muscle and bone, which originates from the ulnar artery 2 cm proximal to the pisiform. This artery runs posteriorly and divides into one branch running distally to supply the pisiform, a muscular branch for the flexor carpi ulnaris and an ascending cutaneous branch. The cutaneous territory can be quite large: the authors' biggest flap was 16 cm long by 6 cm wide. It is the ideal flap for covering the front of the wrist and the ulnar side of the hand (where the flap can reach the proximal phalanx). Its major inconvenience is the shortness of its pedicle.

Lastly, the posterior interosseous flap, independently described by Zancolli and Angrigiani (1986) and Masquelet and Penteado (1987), is a retrograde island flap based on the posterior interosseous vessels. The pedicle is reliable and long, but the size of the flap remains limited and its donor site conspicuous. It remains, however, an ideal flap for the first web.

The radial forearm flap has not dethroned the groin flap of McGregor, which remains the 'king'

of flaps in surgery of the hand. (McGregor & Jackson 1972, Lister et al 1973). Its independent vascular supply, the comfort of the patient, the one surgical operative field, the possibility of performing the operation on ambulatory patients and its versatility in use as a composite flap have all been stressed. These are major advantages in certain circumstances. One must, however, give credit to the groin flap for its great reliability and the inconspicuous donor site. Its use in obese patients is not advisable, but, as has been mentioned, the radial forearm flap suffers from the same disadvantage.

Finally, compared to the free flap the radial forearm island flap has many of the good features of a free flap without the risk inherent in microsurgery. Most of the free flaps (scapular, parascapular, serratus anterior, temporoparietal fascial) have not been used in emergencies and need general anaesthesia, but this is not the case with the lateral arm flap. The texture of the lateral arm flap, the inelasticity of its skin and the thickness of its dermis, as well as its limited size and the cosmetic defect of the donor site, have so far caused the authors to favour the radial forearm flap. An advantage of the lateral arm flap is that it can be raised in a very irregular design, corresponding exactly to the defect. The authors have been lucky not to lose any of their six lateral arm flaps, although in two of the cases the artery was extremely small (less than 1 mm in diameter), necessitating technically exacting microsurgery.

In conclusion the radial forearm island flap finds a place in the indications for cutaneous cover at the level of the hand, especially in emergencies. In addition, its use as a composite flap with a vascularized bone graft allows fewer operative steps in the osteoplastic reconstruction of the thumb. Even though a number of leading centres, including Louisville and Lubljiana, have stressed the value of emergency free flaps, in the authors' experience the radial island forearm flap has not reduced the indications for the groin flap, but has largely taken the already limited place of free flaps.

We would like to acknowledge the help of Mr M. Timmons in kindly reviewing this manuscript.

REFERENCES

Allen E V, 1929 Thrombangiitis obliterans; methods of diagnosis of chronic occlusive arterial lesions distal to the wrist with illustrative cases. American Journal of Medical Science 178–237

Biemer E, Stock W 1983 Total thumb reconstruction: one-stage reconstruction using an osteocutaneous forearm flap. British Journal of Plastic Surgery 36: 52–56

Boorman J G, Brown J A, Sykes P J 1987 Morbidity in the forearm flap donor arm. British Journal of Plastic Surgery 40: 207–212

Braun B J 1977 Les artères de la main. Thèse, Nancy

Braun F M 1984 Le lambeau antébrachial libre ou en îlot en chirurgie de la main. Thèse, Strasbourg, No 6

Braun F M, Hong P, Merle M, van Genechten F, Foucher G 1985 Technique et indications du lambeau antébrachial en chirurgie de la main: à propos de 33 cas. Annales de Chirurgie de la Main 4: 85–97

Colson P, Janvier H 1966 Le degraissance primaire et total des lambeaux d'autoplastie à distance. Annales de Chirurgie Plastique 11: 11–20

Cormack G C, Duncan M J, Lamberty B G H 1986 The blood supply of the bone component of the compound osteocutaneous radial artery forearm flap – an anatomical study. British Journal of Plastic Surgery 39: 173–175

Dellon A L, MacKinnon S E 1984 The pronator quadratus flap. Journal of Hand Surgery 9A: 423

Fatah M F, Davies D M 1984 The radial forearm flap in upper limb reconstruction. Journal of Hand Surgery 9B: 234–238

Fenton O M, Roberts J O 1985 Improving the donor site of the radial forearm flap. British Journal of Plastic Surgery 38: 504–505

Foucher G 1982 Indications du transfert osseux vascularisé en chirurgie de la main. Revue de Chirurgie et Orthopédie II: 38–39

Foucher G, Citron N, Hoang P 1987 Technique and applications of the forearm flap in surgery of the hand. In: Urbaniak J (ed) Microsurgery for major limb reconstruction. C V Mosby, p 256–263

Foucher G, van Genechten F, Merle M, Michon J 1984a A compound radial artery forearm flap in hand surgery: an original modification of the Chinese forearm flap. British Journal of Plastic Surgery 37: 139–148

Foucher G, van Genechten F, Merle M, Michon J 1984b Single-stage thumb reconstruction by a composite forearm island flap. Journal of Hand Surgery, 9B: 245–248

Gelberman R H, Blasingham J E 1981 The timed Allen test. Journal of Trauma 21: 477–479

Gelberman R H, Panagis J S, Taleisnik J, Baumgaertner M 1983 The arterial anatomy of the human carpus Part 1: the extraosseous vascularity. Journal of Hand Surgery 8: 367–375

Gelberman R H, Nunley J A, Koman L A et al 1982 The results of radial and ulnar artery repair in the forearm. Journal of Bone and Joint Surgery 64A: 383–387

Jones B M, O'Brien C J 1985 Acute ischaemia of the hand resulting from elevation of a radial forearm flap. British Journal of Plastic Surgery 38: 396–397

Khashaba A A, McGregor I A 1986 Haemodynamics of the radial forearm flap. British Journal of Plastic Surgery 39: 441–450

Legre R, Kevorkian B, Magalon G 1986 Analyse des sequelles du lambeau antébrachial à pédicule radial: à propos d'une série de 26 cas. Annales de Chirurgie de la Main 5: 208–212

Lin S D, Cai C S, Chiu C C 1984 Venous drainage in the reverse forearm flap. Plastic and Reconstructive Surgery 74: 508–512

Lister G D, McGregor I A, Jackson I T 1973 The groin flap in hand surgery. Injury 4: 229–239

Littler J W 1956 Neurovascular pedicle transfer of tissues in reconstructive surgery of the hand. Journal of Bone and Joint Surgery 38A: 917

Lovie M J, Duncan G M, Glasson D W 1984 The ulnar artery forearm free flap. British Journal of Plastic Surgery 37: 486–492

McGregor A D 1987 The free radial forearm flap – the management of the secondary defect. British Journal of Plastic Surgery 40: 83–85

McGregor I A, Jackson I T 1972 The groin flap. British Journal of Plastic Surgery 25: 3–15

Manchot C 1889 Die Hautarterien des menschlichen Koerpers. F C W Bogel, Leipzig. Republished 1983 Springer-Verlag, Berlin

Masquelet A C, Penteado C V 1987 Le lambeau interosseux postérieur. Annales de Chirurgie de la Main 6: 131–139

Matev I B 1970 Thumb reconstruction after amputation at the metacarpophalangeal joint by bone lengthening: a preliminary report of three cases. Journal of Bone and Joint Surgery 52A: 957–965

Reid C D, Moss A L H 1983 One-stage flap repair with vascularized tendon grafts in dorsal hand injury using the Chinese forearm flap. British Journal of Plastic Surgery 36: 473–479

Schoofs M, Bienfait B, Calfeux N et al 1983 Le lambeau aponeurotique de l'avant-bras. Annales de Chirurgie de la Main 2: 197–201

Small J O, Millar R 1985 The radial artery forearm flap: an anomaly of the radial artery. British Journal of Plastic Surgery 38: 501–503

Song R Y, Gad Y Z, Song Y G et al 1982 The forearm flap. Clinics in Plastic Surgery 9: 21–26

Soutar D S, Tanner N S 1984 The radial forearm flap in the management of soft-tissue injuries of the hand. British Journal of Plastic Surgery 37: 18–26

Timmons M J 1986 The vascular basis of the radial forearm flap. Plastic and Reconstructive Surgery 77: 80–92

Timmons M J, Missotten F E M, Poole M D, Davies D M 1986 Complications of radial forearm flap donor sites. British Journal of Plastic Surgery 39: 176–178

Yang G, Chen B, Gao Y 1981 Forearm free skin flap transplantation. National Medical Journal of China 61: 139

Zancolli E A, Angrigiani C 1986 Colgajo dorsal de antebrazo en 'Isla'. Revista del Associacion Argentina Orthopedico y Traumatico 51: 161–168

5

Distant flaps and reverse dermis flaps

Distant flap transfer is the oldest method of tissue replacement, predating both free graft and free flap repair. Applied to soft-tissue defects of the hand, distant flap techniques have been developed and refined since the start of the 19th century (Chase 1984).

The object is to provide skin which can be used to cover defects of the hand in the acute situation as well as in cold surgery. The early introduction of good quality skin helps to preserve function while providing definitive repair. A flap is required which remains viable when it is used for an acute clinical problem (McGregor 1979); in addition, the flap should be reliable, with a high success rate and a brief attachment phase. Finally, the donor-site defect should be as unobtrusive as possible.

With a greater understanding of the blood supply of skin, culminating in the description of the axial pattern flap by McGregor in 1972, and the perfection of microvascular techniques, the way was paved for free flap transfer by microvascular anastomosis. Although the number of distant flaps performed has declined, they have by no means been eliminated. On the contrary, the discovery of a large number of axial pattern flaps and the recent development of fasciocutaneous and musculocutaneous flaps has made the distant flap method more versatile, simpler and more reliable.

VASCULAR BASIS OF DISTANT FLAPS

There are two types of distant flap, the direct or bridge flap, and the tube pedicle flap. The direct flap has been used successfully in the acute phase of repair, but in order to ensure a viable flap, it has to be raised under strict length-to-breadth ratio restrictions. In general, the length of the flap should be as short as possible and should never exceed the breadth of the base, to avoid the disaster of flap necrosis. In practice, the short length imposes severe constraints on the injured limb, which must be held relatively immobile in a constant position, close to the donor site, for up to 3 weeks until the flap can be divided. The tube pedicle flap has a greater length-to-breadth ratio, affording freer mobility to the attached upper limb. However, it cannot be used for acute hand injuries as it is a delayed flap which needs to be prepared several weeks in advance.

Both types of flap had an unsatisfactory lack of reliability. The incidence and extent of necrosis was variable, and even well-established tube pedicles could necrose when one end was lifted prior to transfer. Gillies, in 1920 pointed out, that flaps in which there was an artery in the base, such as the forehead flap based on the superficial temporal artery, could be cut with a narrow base and would remain viable. Shaw and Payne (1946) described an abdominal flap which could be raised in one stage and tubed to provide cover in hand surgery. This reliable flap was based on the rich vertically orientated blood supply in the lower abdomen, and raised with the superficial inferior epigastric vessels in its base. John Wood performed a similar procedure in 1862, as cited by Khoo Boo-Chai (1977); he later called it a groin flap. It was based on the inferior epigastric vessels and was cut with a greater thickness toward the base of the flap near the vessels. Hynes (1950a) used a rapid tube pedicle method. The flap was raised as a bipedicle strap flap in the lower abdomen, based at the lower end, on the inferior epigastric vessels in the groin. The top end was clamped and fluorescein was injected to test its viability before the one-stage tube pedicle was formed. If the flap did not appear to be viable it could be converted into a standard tube pedicle.

Gradually it became evident that flaps based on known arteries were more robust, and survived with their length considerably greater than the breadth. The deltopectoral flap based on the second and third intercostal arteries was used by McGregor and Jackson (1970) for resurfacing hand defects, and was raised without prior delay. The developing theoretical conflicts were finally crystallized by McGregor in 1972 and McGregor and Morgan in 1973, with the description of the distinction between axial and random pattern flaps. The axial pattern flap is defined as a single-pedicle flap which has an anatomically recognized arteriovenous system running along its long axis. Because of the axial vascular supply, such flaps are freed from many of the restrictions that were traditionally applied to skin flaps. The random pattern flap has no significant dominant arteriovenous blood supply, and is therefore subject to restrictions in flap design: the length should not exceed the breadth (the empirical 1:1 length-to-breadth ratio).

Another advantage of the improved blood supply to an axial pattern flap is that it can be increased in length by adding a random pattern flap on to its distal end. This principle was developed experimentally in the rabbit by Smith in 1973, and confirmed in the human with dye injection studies by McGregor and Morgan (1973). These studies are of fundamental importance in establishing the principles of vascular territories enabling viable axial pattern flaps to be raised on known arteriovenous blood supply. An extension of this phenomenon is the island flap described by Esser (1917), and the neurovascular island flap of Littler (1960), which had the vascular element of its pedicle reduced to an artery and its venae comitantes. As soon as these flaps had been delineated, the way was open for free flap transfer by microvascular anastomosis.

The musculocutaneous flap was first described by Tansini in 1906 and this principle was applied to a distant flap repair by Orticochea in 1972. The skin of this flap is based on the underlying muscle and its vascular pedicle. It has all the properties of an axial pattern flap, and can also be used as an island or free flap.

More recently, the fasciocutaneous flap (Ponten 1981) has been developed as a robust flap which can be raised with a greater length-to-breadth ratio. The blood supply is derived from the rich vascular plexus immediately adjacent to the deep fascia, and for this flap to survive the skin and fascia must therefore be kept in intimate contact and raised in one anatomical entity. Distant fasciocutaneous flaps have been used successfully by Barclay et al (1983).

INDICATIONS FOR FLAP REPAIR

The defect

The need for flap repair depends on the size and site of the defect. In soft-tissue reconstruction the method of repair used should be as simple and economical as possible, in order to diminish the chance of complications and side-effects. This choice in flap surgery is well illustrated by the reconstructive 'ladder' of Nahai and Mathes (1982). Only if simple direct closure, free graft or local flap, in ascending order of complexity, will not provide a repair should a distant or free microvascular flap be considered.

The main indication for a flap is an unsuitable bed for a free skin graft, with exposure of bone, cartilage, tendon or nerve. Flap cover is also indicated in complex injuries, to allow the subsequent reconstruction of underlying bone, joint, nerve or tendon defects.

Available donor sites

If the hand is injured, even though a local flap would be feasible, the introduction of a distant flap would allow greater debridement of the damaged tissue and supply better vascularized tissue. There may be a need to limit further scarring and avoid stiffness from a second wound on the same hand. In a female patient, while function of the hand is vitally important, the surgeon must not ignore perfectly justifiable fears of further disfigurement in a visible area. In these circumstances the relative inconspicuousness of the groin flap donor site has made it the distant flap of choice in hand surgery (Fig. 5.1). Both the quality and quantity of skin required must be carefully evaluated in deciding the choice of flap.

Timing

In the management of a traumatic defect, the general condition of the patient, in addition to the degree of damage to the limb, must be fully assessed. Primary reconstruction of an open hand injury by distant or free flap must only be performed if the patient is in good general shape and able to withstand a prolonged operative procedure. There is no place for a rushed decision without full preoperative assessment and consultation with other specialist colleagues, as necessary. Informed consent, after full discussion of the relevant facts with the patients including degree of donor-site scarring and available alternatives, must be obtained (Winspur 1986).

Most open wounds of the hand can be managed primarily with a moist dressing for several days, so that if the patient is not fit, or if the hand injury is grossly contaminated or infected, delayed primary or secondary repair should be planned. The wound is cleansed, debrided, dressed and inspected again after a few days. Only when the wound is uninfected and clean should distant flap repair be used. If there is any doubt, a further

delay with redressing a few days later may help, or the hand can be wrapped in a temporary split-thickness skin graft. This graft may take and can be replaced later if necessary by a flap repair.

Age of the patient

Distant flap repair entails a two-stage procedure with a period of splintage and fixation in between. There are potential problems with young or nervous patients, where cooperation is difficult to obtain. In older patients the immobility may predispose to stiffness of joints or tendons and contracture formation. No particular age is free of complications and extremes of age do not, per se, rule out distant flap repair (Fig. 5.2). Freedlander et al (1986) reported on a series of groin flaps in patients ranging in age from 18 months to 70 years.

CONTRAINDICATIONS

Donor-site scarring

Scars in a potential donor site must be very carefully evaluated. If there is a scar from a deep wound that might have interfered with the skin blood supply, a flap must not be raised across it. A random pattern flap is very vulnerable to ischaemia from scars because the blood supply depends on the subdermal plexus. A prior-delay procedure with fluorescein testing might clarify the position, but the delay might itself cause skin necrosis.

Malignant disease

When resurfacing after the excision of a malignant condition, if there is any doubt about the completeness of the excision, a distant flap should be used with caution as there is a strong theoretical and practical risk that tumour may be spread into the distant flap donor site.

CHOICE BETWEEN DISTANT OR FREE FLAP

Once a decision has been made that flap cover is required, the choice between a distant flap and a

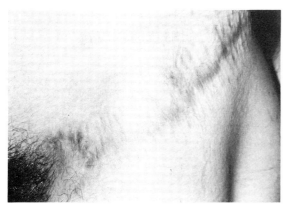

Fig. 5.1 The groin flap donor scar is inconspicuous and easily concealed by clothing.

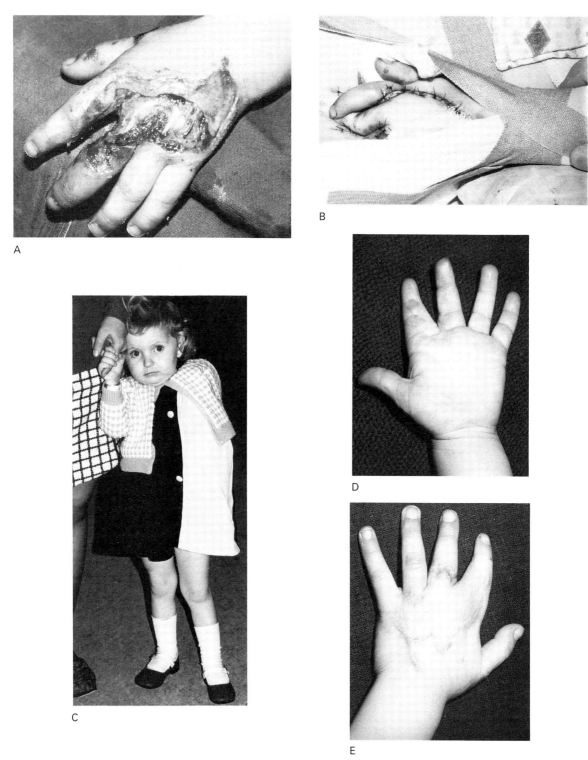

Fig. 5.2 A groin flap used to cover a defect from an electric-bar fire burn in a 3-year-old child. **A** The defect. **B** Groin flap, showing fixation with Elastoplast strapping. **C** The patient tolerated the procedure easily. **D, E** Final result 1 year later, after extensor tendon transfer, thinning and inset of the flap and Z-plasty of the marginal wound.

free flap is often not clear cut. There are certain situations where a free flap has outstanding advantages over all other methods of repair (Mathes & Vasconez 1982), but the decision between the two methods has to be weighed very carefully.

Technical expertise

An obvious prerequisite for microvascular surgery is a thorough knowledge of the necessary technique and the ready availability of all the equipment, including microscope, and back-up facilities including trained staff. Direct distant flap surgery, on the other hand, relies less on technical operative expertise, but more on general reconstructive techniques and good postoperative management. Similarly, this surgery should only be carried out if the surgical and ancillary staff have the necessary experience. One problem of increasing specialization is that the microvascular devotee may decide on a free flap repair when there is an easier, more economical, treatment possible by a traditional flap.

Complex tissue defect

If there is a requirement for composite tissue repair, including skin, bone, joint, etc., and particularly when sensory nerve repair is needed, the free microvascular transfer of an appropriate replacement gives a much more satisfactory and economical repair. The provision of such a repair by the two-stage direct flap followed by further surgery is more cumbersome. However, the microvascular flap is totally dependent on the continuing patency of the anastomoses. If the free flap fails, the total reconstruction may be lost.

Multiple defects

When there are multiple defects on a hand, all requiring flap repair, it is usually technically much easier to use several small direct flaps.

Size of defect

For a large defect, a direct flap of lower abdominal skin or groin flap is probably the treatment of choice. A random pattern flap can be thinned slightly and used as a dermal skin flap (Braithwaite 1950, Colson 1966, see also Chapter 6). This provides thinner, softer, more supple skin and gives a better early result without the need for thinning procedures later. Small defects of non-specialized skin are also most easily made by cross-finger, cross-arm or other direct distant flaps. Medium-sized defects are easily repaired by distant or free flaps. The nature of the tissue defect and flap availability will determine the type of flap required. Fatness in a flap should not nowadays provide great cause for concern, as it can be simply removed by suction lipectomy at a later stage.

No distant flap available

In severe multiple trauma with damage to wide areas of skin, for example burns, or when there is severe damage to the limb and it cannot be moved, it may not be possible to devise a direct flap which can cover the defect. In such cases the free transfer of a distant flap, if available, or a free muscle or fascial flap covered by a skin graft, may be the only solution.

Vascular impairment

When there is very severe injury, particularly crushing or degloving, the severe vascular damage, sometimes extending proximal to the obvious defect, may preclude microvascular free flap repair. A direct flap will bring in a temporarily increased blood flow which might tide the limb over until recovery occurs. Greater problems may ensue at division of the flap in this case. On the other hand, a free microvascular flap on a long pedicle, bridged if necessary by vein grafts, would increase blood supply to the limb.

Patient care and economics

A true comparison of the costs between free and distant flap transfer is difficult to obtain, as many factors have to be taken into account. If the defect is small enough for a cross-finger flap to close it, treatment can be performed as an outpatient procedure, possibly under local anaesthetic, and the operation and accommodation costs are low. A patient with a cross-arm, chest, abdominal or groin flap could also be treated as an outpatient for part of the time during the attachment phase. The transfer of a large amount of skin by direct flap could entail an inpatient stay of 3 weeks or more, and at least two operative stages, which will be extremely costly when bed costs are high. However, the shorter operating time will be less expensive and more cases can be treated in the available theatre time. Free flap transfer is extremely expensive in operating time, but large savings may be made in accommodation costs. There are a few modifications that can be made to speed up the revascularization of a distant flap (see below), which allows earlier division of the flap, thus reducing time spent in hospital.

Postoperative care

The main disadvantage of the two-stage distant flap is the immobility required during the attachment phase. Cross-arm, deltopectoral or upper chest flaps all allow some degree of elevation. The groin flap permits a good range of limb movement but to elevate the hand the patient has to be recumbent. All other considerations being equal, a free flap allows earlier mobilization and elevation of the injured limb, thereby speeding recovery. Unfortunately, the very situations where a direct flap is undesirable, in the older, arthritic or obese patient, are those in which free flap transfer may also be difficult.

BASIC TECHNIQUE

Planning

Thorough preoperative planning is the key to successful distant flap transfer. The object is to provide a viable flap of sufficient size to cover the defect, but the dilemma is that the true extent of the defect may not be fully revealed until it has been made at the time of surgery. In traumatic cases the area of non-viable tissue may be more than expected, while in later reconstructive surgery, after the release of scarred tissue, the defect may expand dramatically. The basic plan must therefore include alternative strategies which

should be considered in advance, preferably before the patient has been premedicated, so that informed consent can be obtained from the patient. Planning with the patient awake also allows a comfortable, relaxed position of donor and recipient sites to be obtained, avoiding stretched or cramped joints.

The flap should be big enough to cover the defect, with a little to spare to allow for the slight swelling and oedema which inevitably occurs after trauma and as a result of surgery. The design must permit the flap to turn into position without excessive tension or twisting, which would interfere with the blood supply. There will inevitably be a need for a bridge segment, which must be taken into account. The best way is to plan and rehearse the procedure using a template of non-expansile material, such as jaconet or polythene sheeting, which can be kept and sterilized to be available during the operation.

Marking

Once the proposed flap has been selected, the outline and relevant anatomical landmarks must be made on the skin with a non-tattooing marker such as Bonney's blue ink. This will aid orientation during the operation and will also give the patient the opportunity to see the extent of donor-site scarring.

The operation

Before the anatomical basis of skin blood supply was properly understood, it was usually recommended that the flap should be raised first to test its viability. However, nowadays it is preferable to establish the defect first. The design of the flap can then be checked and adjusted as necessary, using the sterilized pattern.

It is essential to raise the flap in the correct anatomical plane, which varies with the type of flap being used. A random pattern flap should have a layer of subcutaneous fat included, to avoid damage to the subdermal plexus of vessels. Axial pattern flaps must be elevated to incorporate the axial vessels, and therefore usually have to include the full thickness of subcutaneous fat. Fasciocutaneous and musculocutaneous flaps must be raised deep to fascia or muscle, respectively taking care to ensure that the subcutaneous connections which carry the blood supply are not disrupted. Loose tacking sutures between the skin edge of the flap and the underlying fascia or muscle help to preserve continuity. The donor site and bridge segment should be closed to eliminate open wounds and potential infection, either by direct suture tubing the flap, or with a split-skin graft brought up to line the entire bridge segment.

During the raising and transfer of a flap it must be handled gently to avoid crushing, and protected from dehydration by a covering of saline gauze dressings. After thorough haemostasis the flap and recipient site should be brought into apposition and the flap sutured in place, avoiding tension, torsion or kinking. Closed suction drainage should be used to prevent haematoma formation. Fixation may have to be firm, but if there is a generous lax bridge segment more mobility can be allowed. Dressings and fixation must be carefully applied, leaving a window through which the circulation can be monitored and making sure that there is no pressure on the flap or its base. A major difficulty of direct flap transfer is encountered in the adjustment which have to be made in the early stages. The position is first set up on the operating table, but as the patient wakes or moves, and is transferred back to bed, care is needed to ensure that the flap is not pulled off or kinked. The fixation has to be arranged so that it will stand up to the movements of a restless patient, yet not be so rigid that adjustments in position cannot be made.

Flap viability

During the operation the viability of the flap should be checked from time to time. If at any point the blood supply appears to be compromised, immediate steps must be taken to rectify the situation. If the viability is doubtful when the flap is first raised, it should be laid back in its bed and covered with a warm saline gauze. Any tourniquet or constricting drapes should be removed. After an interval the flap circulation may improve and the operation can proceed. When a flap is sutured in place, if it appears to be too tight, some of the sutures should be removed or the positioning adjusted until the problem is relieved. If the

blood supply is not fully restored, the flap must be completely released and one of the following alternative strategies selected:

1. The operation is treated as a delay stage, the flap is returned to its bed and the recipient site is dressed.
2. The flap can be used to cover part of the defect, supplementing it with a local flap or split-skin graft as appropriate.
3. Another flap should be used.

Postoperative care

Careful monitoring of the flap is essential, particularly in the crucial first day or two. Flap circulation should be inspected regularly by trained nursing staff; any haematoma should be released surgically; external pressure from tight dressings, the patient lying on the flap, or kinking of the bridge segment must be avoided or corrected; prophylactic antibiotics can be used if necessary when an open wound is being covered with a flap; infection should be diagnosed and treated appropriately.

A regular, active regimen of exercises is vital. The help of an experienced physiotherapist is invaluable in helping to encourage the patient to put all joints through as full a range of movement as possible within the constraints of the flap mobility and fixation. These exercises should continue after the pedicle has been divided.

DIVISION

The correct timing of the division of a distant flap is crucial: it must have picked up sufficient blood supply from the recipient site, or it will suffer ischaemia and necrosis. Complications at the attachment site such as infection, mobility or separation of the flap make a longer wait essential. If there is a dominant vessel in the base of the flap, as in an axial flap, peripheral blood supply will be picked up more slowly. A delay before dividing the axial vessel is advisable, particularly if the bridge segment is required to complete the reconstruction.

To some extent the donor site determines the

rate of vascular anastomosis: flaps from an area with a copious blood supply and little subcutaneous fat will take more quickly. An empirical guide is that a cross-arm flap can be divided at 2 weeks, a cross-finger flap at 10 days. Several tests of blood supply are available, the simplest being to clamp the bridge segment with a soft bowel clamp (see Fig. 5.6C). If the flap colour remains unchanged it is viable. A second check is the amount of reactive hyperaemia when the clamp is released after a period of compression. If it is absent the flap has a good attachment. Care is essential in applying this test because of the absence of protective sensation in the flap. The clamp must not be applied too tightly, to avoid crushing the flap. Vital dyes such as fluorescein, injected systemically after a clamp or tourniquet has been applied, are helpful in determining the adequacy of vascularization (McGrath et al 1979).

If there is any doubt about the blood supply a delay procedure, only partially dividing the base, is advisable. Clamping the bridge segment for progressively longer periods can be used as a physiological delay.

At division of the flap, if a significant part of the bridge is to be used to cover the recipient site, it is advisable to delay the formal insetting of the flap to a later stage to avoid a rim of necrosis. Tape sutures applied to approximate the wound edges may avoid the need for a formal inset operation.

Postoperative care

After division, the hand may become oedematous on first mobilizing, and exercises and elevation must continue for a few days. A compression dressing such as Tubigrip should be worn over the flap to prevent oedema. The flap will initially be numb for several months, even if nerve anastomosis has been performed, and it must be protected from excessive trauma, particularly on a load-bearing surface, or trophic damage will occur. Initially the flap will tend to be dry and form crusts at the marginal scar; grease massage will help to keep the skin supple and in good condition. Colour match is usually a problem, as donor areas on the abdomen or groin are usually darker in colour. This can be minimized by avoiding direct exposure to the sun. Applying a sun protection cream to the flap helps if it has to be exposed to the sun.

COMPLICATIONS OF DISTANT FLAPS

Problems can arise from the general complications of surgery, trauma and wound healing, in addition to the specific complications of distant flaps. The most important general complications are the result of the immobility of the attachment phase.

Flap necrosis is the main specific complication, and must be prevented by careful attention to planning and technique as detailed above. Once ischaemia has occurred in a flap it leads to a vicious circle, with further vascular damage due to oedema. Necrosis is then very possible. Vascular insufficiency must be looked for and corrected as soon as it occurs. Venous insufficiency is in some respects more serious – even slight pressure from a dressing or tight sutures can cause venous obstruction, which congests the flap leading to further swelling and tightness and eventually to vascular stasis, arterial obstruction and necrosis. If the blood supply is damaged by technical error at operation, microvascular repair may occasionally be possible, or venous insufficiency can be eased by microvascular anastomosis of a marginal vein to the recipient bed.

Once signs of ischaemia have developed it is usually too late to prevent necrosis, but several measures have been recommended. Elevating a flap with venous insufficiency, or lowering one with arterial insufficiency, may help. Hyperbaric oxygen has been used with some success, but in the absence of controlled clinical studies it is difficult to know how beneficial this is. Vasodilator treatment by alcohol infusion or alpha-blocker drugs have theoretical advantages, but the clinical results are disappointing. Low-molecular weight dextran aids tissue perfusion by decreasing blood viscosity. Cigarette smoking is a potent vasoconstrictor and should not be allowed if the viability of a flap is marginal.

The use of the medicinal leech has had a recent revival (Batchelor et al 1984). These help to decrease congestion in a swollen flap by sucking out blood, but they also release anticoagulant enzymes into the tissues, promoting blood flow and causing the wound to ooze for several hours following application.

Flap skin rarely contracts, but the marginal scar is subject to all the complications of scars. The edge of the flap must be designed to fit along natural crease lines or into the elective lines for skin incision. Long straight edges should be broken up with angular darts, or they can be interrupted by Z-plasty later (see Fig. 5.2D). Small flaps tend to develop a pincushion effect – massage, pressure therapy or marginal Z-plasties all help to relieve this problem.

As the flap retains all the properties of the donor area, poor tissue match is a problem. Distant flaps must be very carefully selected, since the skin will usually be conspicuously different. The best skin repair is to take the anatomically identical tissue from the opposite arm, but this is rarely a solution as it will give severe donor site problems. An abdominal flap is subject to fat deposition if the patient puts on weight. Fat, bulky flaps give cosmetic and functional problems as they tend to slip over the subcutaneous tissue, and thinning them will make them more stable. Hair growth is another problem, and it is important in children to avoid areas which will become hairy later. For example, a low abdominal flap may become hairy at puberty if it is taken from too close to the pubic area.

A scar is inevitable at the donor site, but care should be taken to make it as acceptable as possible and vital structures should not be put at risk. It is essential that an avascular base is not exposed during elevation of a flap if direct closure of the donor site is not possible, otherwise a second flap repair will be required to close the donor defect. The groin flap is popular for hand injuries because of the acceptability of its donor-site scar, in addition to the flap's axial pattern of blood supply (Freedlander et al 1986).

IMPROVEMENTS IN DISTANT FLAP DESIGN

There are two ways in which the design of distant flaps might be improved: increased reliability of the intrinsic blood supply, and increased speed of revascularization of the flap in its bed, so that the attachment phase can be reduced as far as possible.

The development of axial pattern, musculocutaneous and fasciocutaneous flaps has largely satisfied the need for large one-stage flaps that can be safely raised without prior delay. The traditional delay procedure is to be avoided, if possible, as it adds another stage with its own complications and is often counter-productive, especially if the flap becomes infected or bruised. When raised a week later the flap will be stiff and oedematous, and thus may not be able to turn into the defect without tension and kinking.

The flap must remain attached by its pedicle until the blood vessels have linked up sufficiently to support it in its new position. Any manoeuvre that will reliably increase the rate of revascularization will allow the attached phase to be shortened. There are four basic ways in which this can be achieved:

1. An increase in the area of flap attachment
2. An increase in the chance of blood-vessel contact
3. The reverse-dermis flap
4. The crane flap.

Increased area of attachment

The flap must be designed so that it is attached over as wide an area as possible, thus avoiding the need for the bridge segment to be incorporated in the repair. Otherwise a delay will be required, with partial division of the pedicle 1 week prior to detachment. The flap must be sutured accurately edge-to-edge and the free margin closed, if possible by tubing the flap or lining it with a skin graft. Haematoma delays the revascularization phase of flap healing by forming a mechanical barrier to blood-vessel link-up, and must be eliminated by careful haemostasis and closed suction drainage, which gives intimate apposition of the flap to its bed. Shear forces between the flap and its bed must also be avoided by effective fixation. If possible, a tubed flap with a long flexible pedicle is preferred, as the shear forces can be controlled by simple restraint using Elastoplast strapping, to prevent the flap being pulled off its attachment. The broad, short random pattern flap is much more vulnerable to shear forces and there is little leeway for movement. More rigid fixation is essential, with the hand held firmly against the donor site with strapping or bandaging. In practice, the first 48 hours is the crucial period and once fibrin deposition has begun to stick the flap in place, the patient will be warned by the pain if too much pull is exerted.

Increased blood vessel contact

A traditional method of increasing the effectiveness of a tube pedicle attachment is to de-epithelialize the distal segment, which can then be inserted subcutaneously into the recipient site. Deepithelialization, by removing the epidermis and a thin layer of outer dermis, exposes a large number of cut capillaries (Hynes 1950b). The larger area of cut vessels exposed increases the rate of revascularization. If a fasciocutaneous flap is used, a marginal strip of fascia can be inserted in a similar fashion (Thatte et al 1986)

Reverse-dermis flap

The technique of de-epithelialization described above, can be exploited to increase the speed of revascularization of a graft or flap. Hynes, in 1954, used free grafts of de-epithelialized dermis applied upside down, to enhance the take in difficult areas. If there is a larger number of divided blood vessels in the graft, the chance of encounter of vessels needed to revascularize the graft will be greater. Converse et al, in 1975, showed that, in the rat, inosculation of blood vessels can take place within the first 48 hours.

The direct reverse-dermis flap was described by Clodius and Smahel in 1973 as an extension of this principle. The flap was de-epithelialized and attached directly to the bed, with the cut dermis downwards. The flap was divided at 4 weeks, and the exposed vascularized fat was covered with a split-thickness skin graft. Pakiam (1978) reported the use of a reverse-dermis cross-finger flap, which was covered from the outset with a split-thickness skin graft and the pedicle was divided at 14 days. In a series of hand injury defects, Morris (1981) showed that the uptake of blood supply was so rapid in favourable circumstances, that three

reverse-dermis flaps were divided at 7 days with full survival (Fig. 5.3). Another advantage of the method is that the dermal layer, placed deeply, gives a good stable base for the flap and has produced durable cover on palmar surfaces, in contrast to conventional or crane flap repair where the soft fat at the deep aspect causes mobility and is not suitable for load-bearing surfaces. The complication of cyst formation from the buried dermis occurs only infrequently, and any cyst usually absorbs spontaneously. If not it can be excised or marsupialized.

Crane flap

The crane flap principle was first used by Millard in 1969. He proposed that a thick abdominal flap could be used to cover a denuded hand injury; this flap would be separated at 7–10 days by shaving off three-quarters of the thickness of the flap and returning it to the donor site, leaving a thin layer of fascia and subcutaneous fat which could then be grafted with split skin to complete the cover. In pratice it was found that the subcutaneous layer did not easily support a skin graft when first exposed, because of the paucity of blood vessels, but if it is dressed for a few days a skin graft will then take readily.

This technique has the advantages of reducing the time of hand-to-flap immobilization, gives thinner cover free from the complication of hairiness, and leaves a less unsightly donor scar. The method of burying a degloved hand in a subcutaneous pocket and removing it with a layer of viable subcutaneous tissue to be grafted is another example of the crane flap.

The crane flap can be used as a planned procedure (Fig. 5.4). However, if a distant flap develops ischaemia, or the immobilization has to be discontinued for any reason, it can be converted to a crane flap in the hope that there will be enough vascularized tissue to support a skin graft.

REGIONAL FLAPS

The commonly used distant flaps in modern hand surgery are confined to three main donor sites: the trunk, the other arm, and distant flaps from the same hand such as cross-finger or thenar flaps.

Trunk flaps

A flap taken from the anterior upper trunk has the disadvantage of bearing a conspicious donor scar. However, the attached hand is in a relatively elevated position, which helps to reduce oedema and speed mobilization so long as the elbow is not acutely flexed, which might obstruct venous return.

Random pattern flaps from this area are used in resurfacing the thumb or digits, as the quality of skin cover is very good. If the donor site is placed in the axilla, immediately beneath the hair-bearing area, a series of small broad flaps can be raised to cover defects of several fingers. It is preferable to base transversely orientated flaps inferiorly, so that the finger, hand or arm sits down into the flap and contact is reinforced. If the flap is based superiorly the limb will tend to distract from it, due to the pull of gravity, and more complex, firmer fixation will be required. The deltopectoral axial pattern flap based medially on the second and third intercostal perforating arteries provides a large area of skin for hand repair, and can be tubed. The detailed anatomy was described by McGregor and Morgan in 1973. The flap should be raised to include the whole thickness of skin, subcutaneous fat and fascia, stripping the underlying muscle bare. The donor site needs to be grafted.

The lower abdomen has a large area of skin available to provide cover for major defects of the injured limb. Random pattern flaps raised with a thin layer of subcutaneous fat provide good quality cover but the flap length is limited, requiring firm fixation. If the shape and position of the defect allows, inferiorly based flaps are preferable, easing fixation problems (Fig. 5.5).

The hypogastric flap is inferiorly based, with the superficial epigastric vessels as its axial supply. The base is centred over the midpoint of the inguinal ligament, and the flap can be up to 18 cm long, extending upwards and slightly laterally on the lower abdomen. It is raised at the level of Scarpa's fascia. The donor site of a narrow flap can be closed primarily by direct suture, or can be grafted.

The groin flap, described by McGregor and Jackson in 1973, has become the standard distant axial pattern flap for the repair of hand injuries (Fig. 5.6). It is based medially along the line of the groin, on the superficial circumflex iliac vessels. It should be raised at the level of the deep fascia. The flap should not be raised more medially than the inner edge of the sartorius muscle, as the artery is vulnerable to injury at this point where it sends a deep branch beneath the muscle. The donor defect can usually be closed by direct suture, mobilizing the anterior abdominal skin downwards. The groin flap can also be modified to provide an osteocutaneous reconstruction (Reinisch et al 1984) incorporating a segment of iliac crest. For severe degloving injuries, a combined Y-shaped hypogastric and groin flap (Smith 1982) can be used in one stage to cover both surfaces of the upper limb.

The inferiorly based, or the tranverse, rectus abdominis musculocutaneous flap can be used to reconstruct defects of the forearm, and the tensor fascia lata flap has been used as a substitute when the groin flap was not available because of severe burn scars (Nahai & Mathes 1982).

Cross-arm flaps

The opposite arm provides a readily available supply of soft, supple skin ideally suited for the repair of hand and arm defects (see Fig. 5.4). A disadvantage is that the method causes scarring on the undamaged limb, which may not be acceptable. Postoperative care may be difficult with both arms restricted, but by careful design it is usually possible to allow mobility of one hand, and both shoulder joints can be elevated simultaneously. Cross-arm fasciocutaneous flaps, with a longer length-to-breadth ratio, allow more mobility of the attached hand (Dickinson & Roberts 1986). Multiple flaps can be raised if necessary and the upper arm is a convenient site, allowing a comfortable position with the thumb medially and the fingers laterally wrapped round the arm. For fixation, Elastoplast strapping between the two limbs and a sling on each forearm is usually satisfactory (Fig. 5.4C). Reverse-dermis cross-arm flaps allow the attachment phase to be reduced to as little as 1 week (Morris 1981).

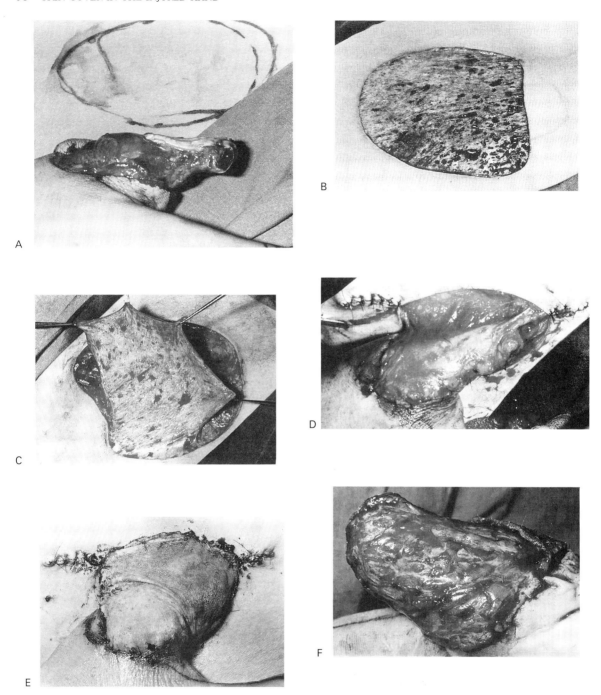

Fig. 5.3 Reverse-dermis flap for thumb reconstruction. **A** Degloved thumb injury wih amputation at the interphalangeal joint level. An abdominal flap is marked out on the lower abdomen. **B** The flap is deepithelialized. **C** The island flap is raised at the periphery, taking care to leave an adequate vascular attachment to the base of the flap. **D** The flap is tubed over the thumb defect and the donor defect is closed by advancing the lower abdominal skin. **E** The reversed flap is then covered by a split-skin graft. **F** One week later the flap can be detached completely from the donor site. An excellent blood supply to the flap can be seen. **G** If necessary, excess soft tissue can be trimmed cautiously and a split-skin graft is then applied. **H** Two weeks later the thumb is virtually healed and the patient was able to return to work. **I** Appearance 2 years later. The tip of the flap has been covered with a sensory flap taken from the radial side of the index finger.

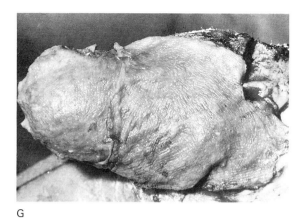

G

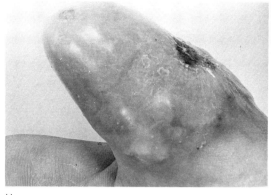

H

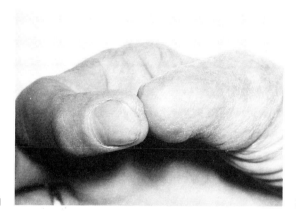

I

Fig. 5.3 Cont'd.

Hand flaps

The cross-finger flap and its modifications are the most commonly used distant flaps in hand repair (Fig. 5.7). A standard random pattern flap is used, raising it at the level of the subcutaneous loose areolar tissue and taking great care not to expose the extensor expansion (Fig. 5.7B). The donor site will require a skin graft. Gaiter strapping holding the fingers in tandem allows good postoperative mobility. This is easily performed under local anaesthetic as an outpatient procedure. The pedicle can be divided at 10 days. The alternative design variations have been described by Tempest (1952) and the reverse-dermis cross-finger flap by Pakiam (1978). Another variation is the cross-finger subcutaneous pedicle flap described by Atasoy (1982).

The thenar flap is not used frequently because of its potential severe complications. The flexion of the finger required to hold the flap in place may cause stiffness, and it is not suitable for the relatively shorter index and little fingers. The donor defect is placed in an important area of the palm and a tender scar would interfere with the power grip.

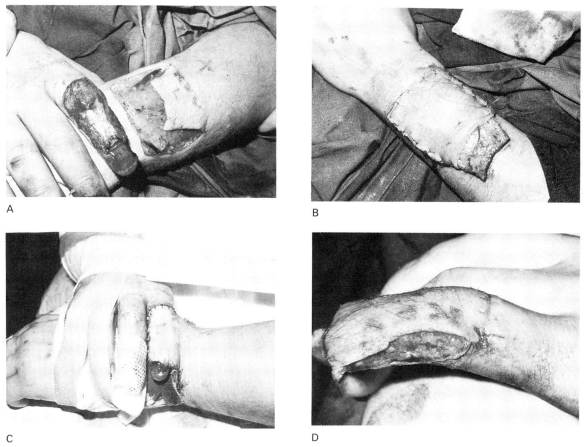

Fig. 5.4 Cross-arm flap illustrating the crane flap principle. **A** The flap is raised in a tattooed area of the forearm, to cover a degloving injury of the right index finger. **B** The donor site and bridge segment are covered with a split-skin graft. **C** The flap is sutured in place and strips of Elastoplast are used for fixation. **D** Two weeks later the bridge is divided. The tattooed skin is excised and discarded and the bed of vascularized subcutaneous fat is covered with a split-skin graft. An alternative if the skin was not tattooed would be to raise the skin and a very thin layer of subcutaneous tissue and return it to the donor site, leaving a layer of vascularized fat to receive a skin graft.

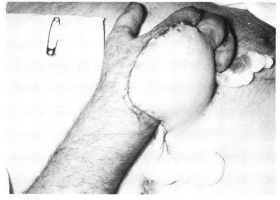

Fig. 5.5 Inferiorly based abdominal flap. The hand sits into the donor site and is held comfortably in place by the Elastoplast loop over the thumb. The donor site is closed by direct advancement of the abdominal wall.

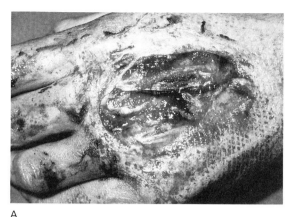

A

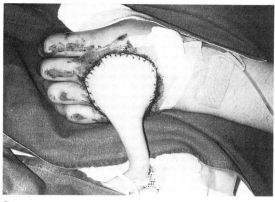

B

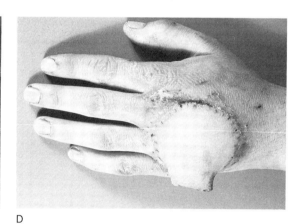

C

D

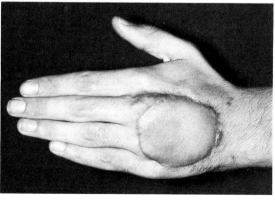

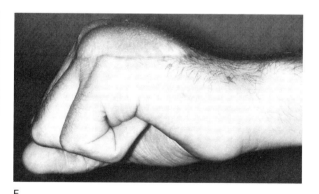

E

F

Fig. 5.6 Groin flap. **A** Defect from a sanding-wheel injury. **B** Groin flap in place. Note the suction drain under the flap and the long pedicle allowing good mobility. **C** A clamp applied to the pedicle at 2 weeks showed good circulation and the flap was divided. **D** The flap stump was sutured directly and early mobilization encouraged. **E, F** The flap was thinned and inset 4 weeks later and the excellent cosmetic and functional result at 6 months is shown.

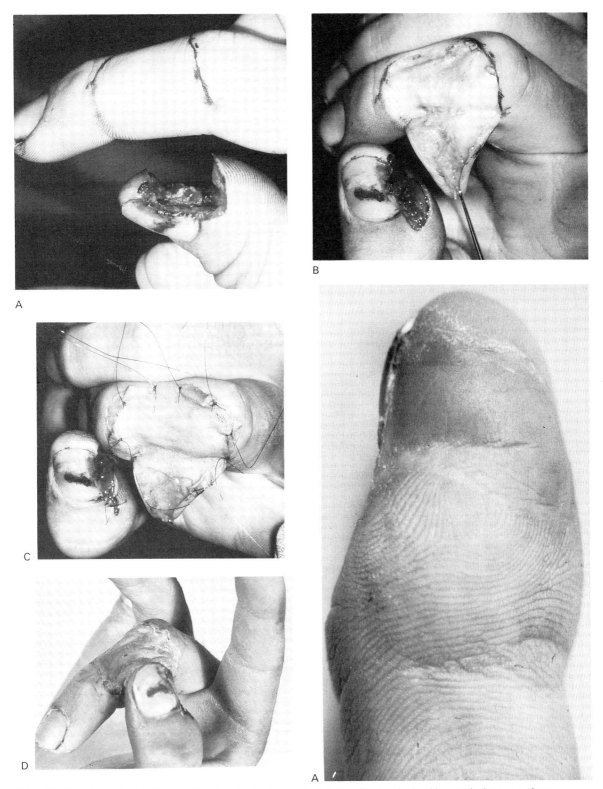

Fig. 5.7 Cross-finger flap. **A** Defect of the thumb with flap marked. **B** The flap is raised, taking particular care to leave paratenon over the extensor tendon. **C** A graft is applied to the donor site and on to the bridge segment. **D** flap in position 2 weeks later, showing the easily maintained comfortable position. The flap is divided under local anaesthetic block of the donor finger, as formal inset is not required of either wound. **E** Result 1 month later.

REFERENCES

Atasoy E 1982 Reversed cross-finger subcutaneous flap. Journal of Hand Surgery 7: 481–483

Barclay T L, Sharpe D T, Chisholm E M 1983 Cross-leg fasciocutaneous flaps. Plastic and Reconstructive Surgery 72: 843–846

Batchelor A G G, Davison P, Sully L 1984 The salvage of congested skin flaps by the application of leeches. British Journal of Plastic Surgery 37: 358–360

Braithwaite F 1950 Preliminary observations on the vascular channels in tube pedicles. British Journal of Plastic Surgery 3: 40–46

Chase R A 1984 The development of tissue transfer in hand surgery. Journal of Hand Surgery 9A: 463–477

Clodius L, Smahel J 1973 The reverse dermal-fat flap: an alternative cross-leg flap. Plastic and Reconstructive Surgery 52: 85–87

Converse J M, Smahel J, Ballantyne D L, Harper A D 1975 Inosculation of vessels of skin graft and host bed: a fortuitous encounter. British Journal of Plastic Surgery 28: 274

Dickinson J C, Roberts A H N 1986 Fasciocutaneous cross-arm flaps in hand reconstruction. Journal of Hand Surgery 11B: 394–398

Esser J F S 1917 Island flaps. New York Medical Journal 106: 264–265

Freedlander E, Dickson W A, McGrouther D A 1986 The present role of the groin flap in hand trauma in the light of a long-term review. Journal of Hand Surgery 11B: 187–190

Gillies H D 1920 Plastic surgery of the face. Hodder and Stoughton, London: p20

Hynes W 1950a The blood vessels in skin tubes and flaps. British Journal of Plastic Surgery 3: 165–175

Hynes W 1950b The rapid transfer of abdominal tubed pedicles. British Journal of Plastic Surgery 3: 202–211

Hynes W 1954 The skin-dermis graft as an alternative to the direct or tubed flap. British Journal of Plastic Surgery 7: 97–107

Khoo Boo-Chai 1977 John Wood and his contributions to plastic surgery: the first groin flap. British Journal of Plastic Surgery 30: 9–13

Littler J W 1960 Neurovascular skin island transfer in reconstructive hand surgery. In: Transactions of the International Society of Plastic Surgeons (Second Congress, London, 1959). E & S Livingstone, Edinburgh: p. 175

McGrath M H, Adelberg D, Finseth F 1979 The intravenous fluorescein test: use in timing of groin flap division. Journal of Hand Surgery 4: 19-22

McGregor I A 1972 Fundamental techniques of plastic surgery, 5th edn. Churchill Livingstone, Edinburgh

McGregor I A 1979 Flap reconstruction in hand surgery: the evolution of presently used methods. Journal of Hand Surgery 4: 1–10

McGregor 1 A, Jackson I T 1970 The extended role of the deltopectoral flap. British Journal of Plastic Surgery 23: 173–185

McGregor I A, Jackson I T 1972 The groin flap. British Journal of Plastic Surgery 25: 3

McGregor I A, Morgan G 1973 Axial and random pattern flaps. British Journal of Plastic Surgery 26: 202-213

Mathes S J, Vasconez L O 1982 In: Green D P (ed) Operative Hand Surgery. Churchill Livingstone, Edinburgh: p 829–855

May J W, Bartlett S P 1981 Staged groin flap in reconstrution of the paediatric hand. Journal of Hand Surgery 6: 163–171

Millard D R 1969 The crane principle for the transport of subcutaneous tissue. Plastic and Reconstructive Surgery 43: 451–462

Morris A M 1981 Rapid skin cover in hand injuries using the reverse-dermis flap. British Journal of Plastic Surgery 34: 194–196

Nahai F and Mathes S J 1982 Upper limb reconstruction. In: Mathes S J, Nahai F (eds) Clinical applications for muscle and musculocutaneous flaps. C V Mosby Company, St Louis: p 624–630

Orticochea M 1972 The musculocutaneous flap method: an immediate and heroic substitute for the method of delay. British Journal of Plastic Surgery 25: 106–110

Pakiam I A 1978 The reversed dermis flap. British Journal of Plastic Surgery 31: 131–135

Ponten B 1981 The fasciocutaneous flap: its use in soft-tissue defects of the lower limb. British Journal of Plastic Surgery 34: 215–220

Reinisch J F, Winters R, Puckett C L 1984 The use of the osteocutaneous groin flap in gunshot wounds of the hand. Journal of Hand Surgery 9A: 12–17

Shaw D T, Payne R N 1946 One-stage tubed abdominal flaps. Single-pedicle tubes. Surgery, Gynaecology and Obstetrics 83: 205-209

Smith P J 1973 The vascular basis of axial pattern flaps. British Journal of Plastic Surgery 26: 150–157

Smith P J 1982 The Y-shaped hypogastric-groin flap. Hand 14: 263–270

Tansini I 1906 Sopra il mio nuovo processo di amputazione della mamella. Giornale Italiano di Medicina 57: 141

Tempest M N 1952 Cross-finger flaps in the treatment of injuries to the finger tip. Plastic and Reconstructive Surgery 9: 205–222

Thatte R L, Yelicar A D, Chhajlani P, Thatte M R 1986 Successful detachment of cross-leg fasciocutaneous flaps on the tenth day: a report of 10 cases. British Journal of Plastic Surgery 39: 491–497

Winspur I 1986 Complications following secondary reconstructive procedures of skin and subcutaneous tissue. In: Boswick J A (ed) Complications in hand surgery. W B Saunders Company, Philadelphia: p 303

The flap graft

Flap cover is frequently required in traumatic injuries involving tissue loss, such as burns or degloving injuries, and, more rarely, after tumour ablation. The majority of defects occur on the dorsum of the hand and fingers, and a flap is used either to obtain epithelial cover over bone, tendon or nerve, where a skin graft might not survive, or to provide suitable cover under which tendon grafting or other reconstructive surgery can be performed.

PRINCIPLES OF FLAP COVER

The hand has both sensation and movement. Both of these features must be preserved in any reconstructive work, and aesthetic and functional considerations go together. Stiffness is to be avoided at all costs in hand surgery, through the prevention of scarring, contracture and infection. Sensation can be provided by spontaneous re-innervation of the flap from local tissues, or by deliberate means such as nerve anastomoses or island flaps. The principles of adequate early surgical debridement are well understood, as are the indications for flap cover. Problems arise, however, in the type of flap to be chosen. On the dorsum of the hand a flap needs to be thin, very pliable, and should not require the hand to be immobilized in any position other than a functional one. Furthermore, the hand needs to be elevated to limit oedema formation. Common examples include the groin flap, the axillary flap, the inframammary flap and, more recently, the reverse radial forearm flap and free flaps. All these flaps suffer from being bulky, even in otherwise

thin patients. The dual problems of repeated surgical thinnings and limitation of mobility are familiar to most hand surgeons. One of the best ways to circumvent the limitations of these different flaps is to use the 'flap graft'.

SURGICAL TECHNIQUE

The flap graft was first described by Colson and Janvier (1966) and is well suited for hand reconstruction. It consists of a flap of skin based on the dermal blood supply. Typically the donor area consists of the thin skin on the volar surface of the opposite arm, although other sites have been used, including the groin. Having placed the affected hand in a comfortable position, two incisions are made in the donor area in such way that the affected part can be passed beneath the intervening skin (Fig. 6.1). To cover a finger, for example, the incisions are twice the breadth of the finger. The flap is then undermined at the level of the

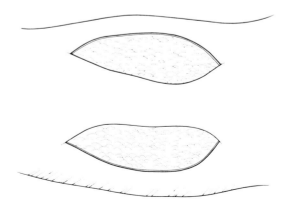

Fig. 6.1 Incisions to raise a dermal flap graft.

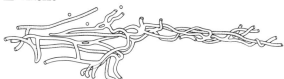

Fig. 6.4 Schematic representation of the papillary plexus.

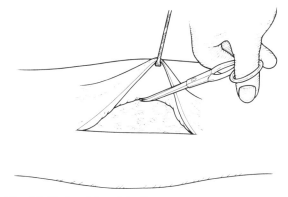

Fig. 6.2 Undermining of the flap.

dermis (Fig. 6.2), and the finger is inserted into the pocket which has been created (Fig. 6.3). Where several fingers need to be covered, a single flap can be used. It is important to ensure that tension in the flap is avoided by making the incisions sufficiently long. This is particularly true where bony protuberances such as the metacarpophalangeal joints are to be covered. The two ends of the flap are sutured to the defect and the arms are strapped together, or secured with slings as described by Chapman (1986). After an interval of approximately 18 days, the pedicles of flap are divided and inset into the edges of the defect. The secondary defect is closed directly or grafted. Early mobilization of the finger or hand can be carried out, and further reconstructive work such as tendon grafting may be performed when the induration has settled, typically after a further 2 months.

ANATOMY

Much work has been carried out in recent years on the blood supply of skin flaps. Nakajima et al (1986) classified skin flaps into five main categories, from 'cutaneous flaps' to 'musculocutaneous flaps', and Cormack and Lamberty (1984) analysed in great detail the patterns of vascular supply in fasciocutaneous flaps. All authors agree that

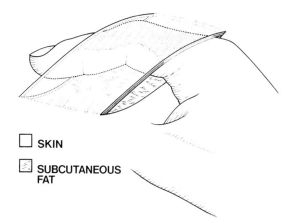

☐ SKIN

☒ SUBCUTANEOUS FAT

Fig. 6.3 Finger in situ beneath flap.

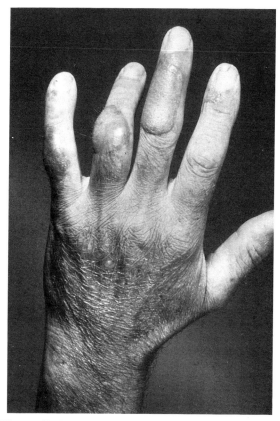

Fig. 6.5 End result 1 year post-injury in a patient whose middle, ring and little fingers have been resurfaced with flap grafts, which required no thinning.

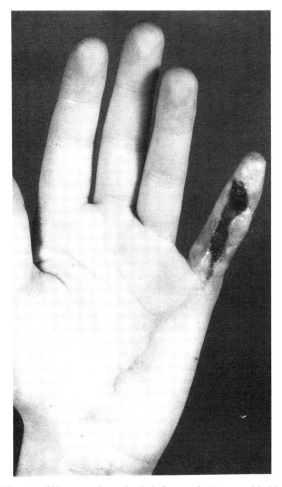

Fig. 6.6 Skin necrosis on the little finger of a 15-year-old girl following insertion of a silastic rod.

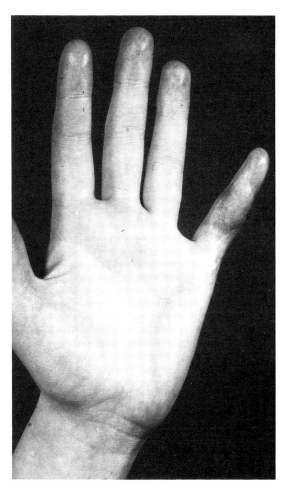

Fig. 6.7 Following resurfacing with a flap graft taken from the groin. No thinning was necessary, and tendon and nerve reconstruction was later completed.

there is a common end-point of the blood supply to the skin, namely the horizontal plexus of the papillary dermis.

This plexus of vessels was carefully studied by Yen and Braverman (1976), who demonstrated that there are three important plexuses in the dermis: a horizontal network in the papillary dermis out of which the capillary loops arise, and individual plexuses around hair follicles and eccrine sweat glands. The bulk of this micro-circulation resides in the papillary plexus, which consists of terminal arterioles, capillaries and postcapillary venules. These venules are the vessels most frequently encountered on microscopic analysis of the skin, and the flow into them from the arterioles is normally controlled by the precapillary sphincter. Direct connections between the arteriolar and venous plexuses in the papillary dermis bypass the capillary bed (Fig. 6.4).

While the author is not aware of any work to show the respective proportion of the circulation through the dermis and subcutaneous fat, it is generally accepted that the fat is poorly supplied by specific vessels. It would appear, therefore, that there is no reason why 'random' pattern flaps should include the subcutaneous fat, as it will not help the viability of the flap and may be a drain on its vascular supply. The viability of the flap graft is therefore entirely dependent upon the horizontal plexus, which has a rich blood supply that can be augmented by control of the postcapillary sphincters.

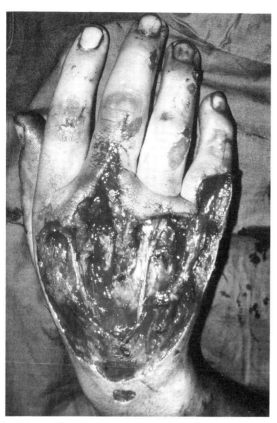

Fig. 6.8 Skin was lost from the dorsum of the hand due to a 'roll-over' motor accident.

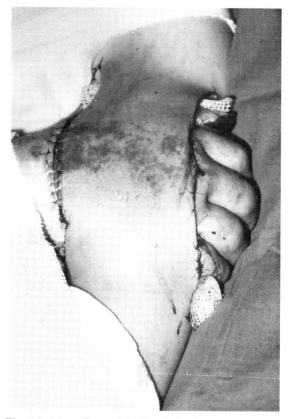

Fig. 6.9 A large flap graft in place. There is some discoloration of the centre of the flap, but this recovered.

ILLUSTRATIVE CASES

Figure 6.5 shows the result following flap cover on the middle, ring and little fingers of a 46-year-old man. No thinning of the flaps has been required.

Figure 6.6 shows an area of skin necrosis on the little finger of a 15-year-old girl following insertion of a silastic rod for flexor tendon reconstruction. This was replaced with a flap graft (Fig. 6.7), allowing the tendon and nerve reconstruction to be completed. The donor site for the flap graft in this case was the groin.

The skin loss shown in Fig. 6.8 occurred in a road accident. This was debrided under general anaesthesia and covered with a split-skin graft as a biological dressing. Three days later, the patient was given a cross-arm dermal flap to cover the defect. This flap was considerably larger than those previously used, and the central part of the

flap, which was also the area under maximum tension, was of suspect viability (Fig. 6.9). By 3 weeks it had recovered, and the flap was

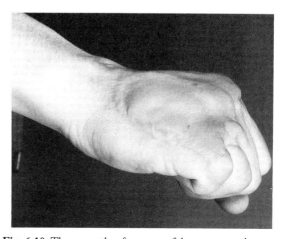

Fig. 6.10 Three months after successful extensor tendon grafting.

divided and inset. At 3 months the patient successfully underwent extensor tendon reconstruction beneath the flap, which remained soft and pliable, and no further treatment was required (Fig. 6.10).

The dermal flap has proved to be a consistently sound method of reconstruction for patients with skin loss over the dorsum of the hand or fingers. While the initial indication for its use was thought to be mainly in electrical burns of the hand or fingers (Colson et al 1967), it has been used in a wide variety of conditions. There is one major problem with the technique, namely the unsightly donor-site scar when the flap is taken from the arm. The patient illustrated in Figs 6.8–6.10 was not in the least concerned by its appearance and refused revisional surgery.

REFERENCES

Chapman C 1986 The immobilisation of cross-arm flaps. British Journal of Plastic Surgery 39: 260–261
Colson P, Janvier H 1966 Le degraissage primaire et total des lambeaux d'autoplastie a distance. Annales de Chirurgie Plastique 11: 11–20
Colson P, Houot R, Gangolphe M et al 1967 Utilisation des lambeaux dégraissés (Lambeaux – Greffes) en chirurgie reparatrice de la main. Annales de Chirurgie Plastique 12: 298–310
Cormack G C, Lamberty B G H 1984 A classification of fascio-cutaneous flaps according to their pattern of vascularisation. British Journal of Plastic Surgery 37: 80–87
Nakajima H, Fujino T, Adachi S 1986 A new concept of vascular supply to the skin and classification of skin flaps according to their vascularization. Annals of Plastic Surgery 16: 1–17
Yen A, Braverman I 1976 Ultrastructure of the human dermal microcirculation : the horizontal plexus of the papillary dermis. Journal of Investigative Dermatology 66: 3 131–142

David M. Evans and David Gault

General principles of free tissue transfer

The advent of free tissue transfer by microvascular techniques has streamlined the treatment of many patients, and introduced possibilities that did not exist before (Daniel & Taylor 1973). Nevertheless, there are occasions when older techniques of major skin replacement are applicable, and they should always be considered (Wood & Irons 1983).

The principal advantage of free tissue transfer lies in the possibility of completing the entire reconstruction in one stage, thus shortening the treatment period, avoiding multiple anaesthetics, and reducing the mental stress on the patient. It is easier to contemplate and endure one burst of treatment than repeated ones; nevertheless, these advantages are not always realized, since the primary healing time is often longer than expected, secondary procedures are frequently required, and loss of a free flap, which will occasionally occur, is likely to be total and catastrophic.

In this chapter general indications for free tissue transfer will be considered, followed by technical aspects common to all such cases.

GENERAL INDICATIONS

Distant flap cover is required when the simple possibilities of a free skin graft or local flap are not applicable (see Chapters 2 & 3). Many factors have to be taken into account when making this choice. Not only must the size, depth and contents of the defect be considered, but also the patient's age and general condition, the existence of adverse circumstances such as diabetes, irradiation and pre-existing infection, and the require-ment for additional reconstructive procedures at the same time or later. A free tissue transfer may be indicated under the following circumstances:

1. An extensive skin and subcutaneous tissue defect involving several areas of the hand and fore-arm. The wish to avoid immobilization and de-pendency might lead to the choice of a free flap rather than a large groin flap or combined groin, epigastric or abdominal flap (McGregor & Jackson 1972, Smith 1982).

2. A skin defect overlying structures which also need replacement, particularly tendon, bone or joint. Here a composite flap carrying other tissues with their vascularity may be appropriate.

3. A skin defect in an important tactile area, in which restoration of good sensation in the flap is necessary.

4. Skin loss in the first web space too large to cover with a local skin flap.

Naturally there are alternative methods for all of these: the relative indications are discussed in detail elsewhere in the book.

Free tissue transfer is a surgical undertaking in which every detail of the operation has to be right – one missing link can mean total failure. There-fore, to achieve a high success rate each case demands careful planning, good teamwork and flawless execution.

PLANNING

The first stage of planning is the decision to use a free flap, having excluded all other possible methods. This should be based on clearly perceived advantages. The procedure makes large demands in time and effort from the whole team, and it should be clear to all why they are required to make that effort. However, as techniques become more commonplace and take less time, with a lower complication rate, attitudes change and the balance of choice becomes more weighted in favour of the new technique.

The next choice concerns the tissue or tissues best suited to the particular reconstructive problem, and where that tissue can be taken with minimal donor-site problems (Fig. 7.1). For simple resurfacing, a skin flap gives the best texture, colour and lack of contractile tendency, but most

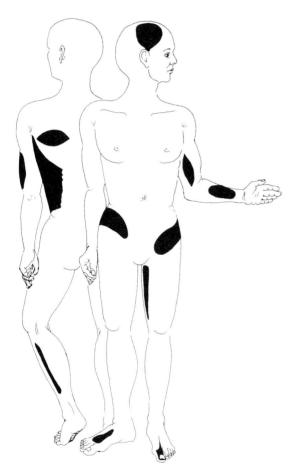

Fig. 7.1 Diagram showing most of the free flap donor sites available for use in the hand and upper limb. From above downwards they are: temporoparietal fascia, scapular, latissimus dorsi, medial arm, lateral arm, radial forearm, deep circumflex iliac, groin, gracilis, fibula, dorsalis pedis and wraparound big toe.

free skin flaps carry too much subcutaneous fat, particularly for use in the palm, where fat makes the skin too mobile and occupies space which should be available for a grasped object. For small defects the dorsalis pedis flap has less subcutaneous fat than most donor sites (McCraw & Furlow 1975), but the adherent graft on the dorsum of the foot can be troublesome. The lateral arm flap (Katsaros et al 1984, see also Chapter 8) is acceptable in thin subjects, but does carry its share of fat and the medial arm flap may prove superior from this point of view (Dolmans et al 1979). The radial forearm flap is a good competitor (see Chapter 4) and if not available as a local island flap, can be taken from the opposite forearm as a free flap.

To avoid the inclusion of subcutaneous fat a free transfer of muscle or fascia resurfaced with a free skin graft may be chosen. Temporoparietal fascia can be used in this way, and can wrap around fingers and through web spaces (Upton et al 1986, see also Chapter 9); for large defects the latissimus dorsi muscle provides excellent reconstructive material, wrapping around both surfaces of the hand if necessary. Initially the muscle is bulky, although the outer surface and the section above the entry of the pedicle can be trimmed (Godina 1987, Rowsell et al 1986, Tobin et al 1981), and denervation of the muscle results in some subsequent atrophy, although this is variable. Later thinning is difficult, usually involving shaving and regrafting, in contrast to a skin flap which can be thinned by liposuction or surgical excision of fat. Vascularized muscle or fascia takes a free skin graft well, particularly an unexpanded mesh graft, but the resulting surface is never as soft and supple as that of a skin flap, and there may be some tendency to contract, particularly in the palm and web spaces. Thick split-skin grafts and full-thickness (Wolfe) grafts convey some advantage in this respect, and are also better cosmetically. On the dorsum of the hand the surface of a mature grafted fascial flap should be ideal. Any tendency to hypertrophy of the graft and scars calls for the use of a compression glove.

For very large defects involving areas of the forearm as well as the hand a myocutaneous flap may be chosen, usually the latissimus dorsi flap, but the problem of bulk is compounded by the presence of both muscle and subcutaneous fat.

Free tissue transfer comes into its own when other deep tissues are also required. Loss of skin and all extensor tendons on the dorsum of the hand is a good indication for this, being the only way of restoring independent tendon and skin function in one stage. Small defects with limited loss of one or two tendons can be treated by simple skin grafting, and a suprising amount of active extension can be restored by a tenodesis effect. This is not as good as full finger movement independent of wrist position, which should be the aim of treatment. A composite flap of skin with four long extensor tendons can be taken from the dorsum of the foot (dorsalis pedis flap), and this procedure will be described (see Chapter 10).

The use of muscle as a soft-tissue repair has been mentioned, but it may also be reinnervated and used to replace missing major muscle groups. Limited muscle loss is usually better dealt with by tendon transfer, and free muscle transfer is limited to cases in which adjacent muscles are not available for transfer. This is unfortunate, since such cases have usually undergone major trauma, with damage to distal tendon gliding mechanisms and skeletal components, and with only short scarred tendon ends to attach the muscle to distally. This limits the potential success of the procedure. The technical process of moving a muscle as a free transfer on a neurovascular pedicle is not difficult, and good contractility can be expected because the motor nerve repair can be accomplished without tension, and close to the muscle in most circumstances. If this were indicated in less challenging cases better results could be expected, although it has been observed that a substantial decrease in muscle bulk and strength is to be expected following muscle transplantation (Terzis et al 1978); Manktelow et al (1984) has shown, however, that useful results can be achieved.

Extensive skin and bone loss is not common in the hand and can usually be dealt with by independent soft-tissue cover over a free cortico-cancellous bone graft. The complexity and morbidity of a deep circumflex iliac flap with iliac crest and overlying skin would seldom be justified for this indication, but might occasionally be required in the forearm, and similarly the fibular osteocutaneous free flap might very rarely be used. Small pieces of distal phalanx are included with composite partial free toe transfers and wrap-around flaps (Morrison et al 1980), and are useful both to provide skeletal support for the nail and fingertip, and to attach to the distal end of a free bone graft when used for the main skeletal support of the reconstructed digit. It has been found that a free bone graft placed between two vascular bones undergoes far less resorption, this being a potential problem of the wraparound technique of digital reconstruction.

Free vascularized toe-joint transfer has a limited place in digital reconstructive surgery, being indicated in a young patient in whom prosthetic arthroplasty is excluded by dorsal skin and extensor tendon damage; where arthrodesis is undesirable because of patient preference; where multiple digits are involved; and when epiphyses are still open, since this type of transfer can give additional growth to the finger (Foucher et al 1986). The transfer includes skin, extensor tendon and PIP joint, and can include the fibro-osseous canal of the flexor tendons if necessary. It is difficult to avoid a flexed resting posture for the transferred joint, because of anatomical differences and difficulty in intrinsic reconstruction, but a stable range of 30°–50° can be achieved.

When important tactile areas are resurfaced it is important to reinnervate the flap (Coleman & Jurkiewicz 1984, Mathes & Buchanan 1979, May et al 1977). When skin only is used in a flap repair there is some reinnervation from the edges and the underlying bed, but this is not good enough on the fingertips and is barely adequate for the palm. If a muscle or myocutaneous flap is used there is no spontaneous sensory reinnervation. For finger or thumb pulp reconstruction a free neurovascular flap can be taken from the lateral pulp of the big toe, with or without the nail and underlying bone. For small defects there are, of course, alternatives available in the form of pedicle or island flaps within the hand, but for the right indications free toe pulp transfers are excellent, and have the advantage of correct orientation of the sensory reinnervation. Larger areas of innervated skin can be replaced by using the dorsalis pedis flap carrying the superficial peroneal nerve, which is then anastomosed to a local available sensory nerve (Daniel et al 1976). The quality of sensory recovery is limited by the relative sparsity of sensory endings in the dorsum of the foot, and the fact that most of the axons in the superficial peroneal nerve pass through the flap and emerge distally in the dorsal sensory nerves to the toes, which are divided. The tensor fascia lata myocutaneous flap can be reinnervated using the lateral cutaneous nerve of the thigh, but it is a bulky flap for use in the hand.

Having decided which free tissue transfer to use and what to include, the surgeon should set time aside for detailed planning, since this is the best way to limit unforeseen problems which can threaten the success of the procedure. First a 'tissue diagnosis' should be made, measuring or estimating the extent of the defect of each tissue involved, and the spatial relationship of missing areas of adjacent tissues. This may be a matter of simple measurement, or in a severely contracted wound may require the measurement of existing landmarks and comparing them with the intact opposite limb. Such measurements can be confirmed during surgery when the cicatricial scar has been excised. A 20–30% allowance for natural elastic recoil should always be made, since the swelling attendant upon surgery usually prevents the skin from re-expanding to its original dimensions without jeopardizing the circulation.

Next the position and length of the pedicle have to be considered, and its relationship to available vessels in the recipient area. This is a most important part of planning. A small discrepancy in the position or angle of approach of the pedicle can result in unexpected difficulty in the anastomoses. If necessary, vein grafts can be used (Biemer 1977), but it is better to plan their use from the start and have them available in advance of the anastomosis than to have to use them unexpectedly. Although the number of anastomoses is increased by the use of vein grafts, time is normally saved when they are planned from the start, and there are no wasted minutes of indecision or fruitless attempts at anastomosis under adverse conditions (Chow et al 1982). If an innervated flap is planned, similar consideration has to be given to the length and position of the sensory nerves to be repaired.

Finally the logistics of the operation have to be planned. For most transfers to the upper limb the patient is supine throughout the procedure, but latissimus dorsi or scapular flaps require a lateral position during raising, and the patient may need to be turned once, or even twice. This is in fact good for the patient, but the anaesthetist needs to be prepared. The operation is streamlined if two teams can work simultaneously to prepare the flap and the recipient area, and later to repair the donor defect while the reconstruction is completed. This needs careful planning and timing. It is important to allow time for the flap to perfuse in its old position, after dissection but prior to transfer, both to confirm that the circulation within the flap is intact and to allow homeostasis to be re-established up to the time at which the vessels are divided. This limits the ischaemic changes within the flap that could interfere with the re-establishment of circulation.

ANAESTHESIA

Although it is possible to transfer free flaps under regional or spinal anaesthesia, general anaesthesia is more usual because of the multiple operative sites, and the length of time required which might make the procedure an unacceptable ordeal. The anaesthetist should be familiar with the special anaesthetic demands of these patients. Bounding peripheral perfusion must be maintained, to generate rapid flap perfusion on release of the vascular clamps, with good anastomotic flow helping to secure a low occlusion rate. This is achieved by the obsessive maintenance of body temperature through insulation and the use of a heated ripple mattress, and the maintenance of a high circulating volume through colloid, crystalloid and if necessary blood transfusion coupled with alpha-adrenergic blockade to dilate the vascular bed (Awwad et al 1983a,b). These two objectives have to be kept in mind from the start of the anaesthetic; if any ground is lost in either respect it is difficult to regain a favourable position, and this, coupled with preoperative smoking (which should be forbidden), is the most likely cause of arterial spasm, with failure of flap perfusion on release of the clamps (Nolan et al 1985).

A urethral catheter is helpful in monitoring fluid balance, and prevents a full bladder at the end of the procedure which leads to a restless patient and may also cause reflex vascular changes. During long procedures special care must be taken of pressure areas, peripheral nerves and the eyes.

THE OPERATION

The detailed technique of raising individual flaps is discussed under the various donor areas. Preparation of the recipient area involves the excision of diseased, dead or scarred tissue, and the re-establishment of anatomical relationships, confirmation of the preoperative tissue diagnosis, and, if necessary, adjustment of the design-plan of the flap. Underlying structures to be reconstructed have to be prepared and labelled if necessary, and the recipient vessels dissected out and prepared, with confirmation of patency. They should not be divided or clamped until the time of anastomosis. This stage may be completed under tourniquet control, but this should be released when the area is prepared, and the remaining steps of the operation completed without tourniquet.

It is most important to suture the flap vessels to healthy recipient vessels, outside the zone of trauma and surrounded by healthy undamaged tissue. There is no shortage of arteries in the hand and forearm (Coleman & Anson 1961), and deep or superficial venous systems can be used for drainage. In the severely traumatized or congenitally abnormal limb, however, there may not be abundant vessels, and the preoperative planning must be relied on to guide the vascular dissection. In the hand the most versatile site for vascular anastomosis is in the region of the anatomical snuffbox, where the cephalic vein crosses the radial artery, and venae comitantes are also available. The arterial anastomosis should be done end-to-side, as this preserves existing arterial input to the hand, and also provides safer vascular supply to the flap (Albertengo et al 1981, Godina 1979, Ikuta et al 1975). If a side hole is cut in an artery, the contraction of circular muscle which takes place following vessel trauma has the effect of opening the hole wider, thus increasing the outflow of blood from the artery (Fig. 7.2);

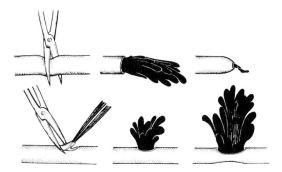

Fig. 7.2 Illustration of the principle underlying end-to-side arterial anastomosis. If an artery is divided transversely the initial gush diminishes with circular muscle contraction. By contrast, following the creation of a sidehole this increases bleeding.

traumatic side holes in arteries have a tendency to bleed profusely, and this can be harnessed with end-to-side anastomosis, allowing the artery to bleed into the flap. Good exposure of the artery is important, and in the snuffbox the radial artery has to be dissected freely, so that it can be easily delivered to the wound surface for anastomosis, with ample room for clamps. It is useful to be able to pass a smooth instrument such as the wide end of a Howarth's elevator beneath the artery during anastomosis, but the artery must not be subjected to traction beyond the loose elastic state. The vein can be repaired end-to-side if the vessels lie more easily, but there is no particular advantage from the haemodynamic point of view, and end-to-end anastomosis is usually more straightforward. If necessary, additional length of vein can be made available by dissecting the vein distally and transposing it into the desired position. The pedicle may be passed through a tunnel to the site of anastomosis, but this must be prepared to allow free introduction of the pedicle with no kinking or tension, and an ample size of tunnel to accommodate the pedicle and allow for swelling. Even for a thin pedicle it should always be possible to pass a finger through the tunnel with ease.

Microvascular repair

Once the basic technique of microvascular repair has been acquired, the actual suturing of the vessels should be the simplest and most relaxed phase of the operation. To achieve this ideal state, however, demands meticulous preparation. Success can only be expected if the anastomosis is between healthy vessels in a readily accessible situation, with no tension and in a well-perfused patient. The planning of the flap and recipient area contributes much to this, but it is also important not to rush the critical stage of transfer of the flap from donor to recipient area, and preparation of the vessels for anastomosis.

When the flap is introduced to the recipient area the fit should be checked, and the correct placing and length of the pedicle confirmed. The flap should then be anchored in place to ensure stability during and after vessel repair, taking care to protect the loose pedicle from damage or entrapment. If bone fixation or complicated repair of deep structures are required these are usually best completed before vessel anastomosis. Great care is required if the pedicle has to be tunnelled to the anastomotic site. It should be pulled through gently with a suture attached to a safe accompanying structure or connective tissue (not a vessel or a clamp), and a trailing stitch should be left to allow retrieval of the pedicle if a problem arises. Smooth passage through the tunnel is facilitated by enclosure of the pedicle in the separated finger of a rubber glove with a hole in the end for the traction stitch (Fig. 7.3). Without this precaution part of the pedicle may become snagged, or a clamp, ligaclip or suture may catch on an irregularity in the tunnel. It is always worth double-checking that there is no twisting or kinking of the pedicle. If the recipient vessels have been well prepared, the operating microscope is now introduced and the position of the vessels is checked. Final preparation of the flap vessels consists of gentle dilatation with smooth vessel dilators (the only instrument that should come into contact with the vascular endothelium).

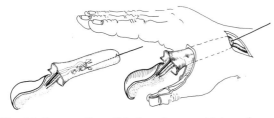

Fig. 7.3 Passage of a pedicle through a tunnel is hazardous, and is made easier by enclosing the pedicle in a glove finger, which is split and removed once the pedicle is in place.

Instrumentation can be simplified by using two pairs of vessel dilators as needle holders and tissue forceps as well as for handling vessels, the only other instrument required being sharp curved microscissors. The vessel lumen is then irrigated with heparinized Hartmann's solution (1 ml of 1:1000 per 500 ml) (Harashino & Buncke 1975, Buchler et al 1977). If the vessels have been clamped with gentle (less than 50 gm) microvascular clamps, a useful measure to assist identification, these should be loosened and the blood washed out. Loose adventitia should be trimmed to prevent fronds being trapped in the anastomosis, and the cut end of each vessel should be checked to ensure that it is cleanly cut, with no crushing. If necessary it should be cut back further.

Attention is turned to the recipient vessels. If one is likely to conceal the other following anastomosis, the least accessible should be repaired first; if not, it is better to anastomose the vein first, so that the clamps can be removed, thus limiting endothelial damage, without the bleeding and congestion that would result from prior release of the artery. For end-to-end anastomosis the vein is prepared in the same way as the vessels in the pedicle; the vessels should be divided with allowance for elastic recoil, so that a tension-free anastomosis can be accomplished. For large vessels 8/0 nylon is fine enough, provided that a fine needle is used, but 10/0 nylon can be used safely if the surgeon prefers. Troublesome leakage from the vein is unusual, but accurate apposition is important, with a sufficient number of sutures to maintain it as the vessels fill and dilate. Vessels of unequal size need great care in the placing of sutures. It helps to cut the smaller vessel slightly obliquely, but not too much, although adaptation is achieved mainly through the even distribution of sutures. The order of suture placement is a matter of personal preference and training. If access is limited, the furthest sutures should be placed first and successive sutures inserted from behind forwards on each side of the original stitch (Harris et al 1981). This avoids the need to turn the vessels in order to suture the back wall, but demands good judgement in the placing of sutures to include an equal proportion of the circumference of the two vessels in each stitch. Knots must be safely tied, with two turns on the first of three throws. During suturing all vessels, including nearby branches, should be held in appropriately gentle vascular clamps to avoid blood leakage, and it is similarly important to have good haemostasis in the surrounding field before starting. If this is impossible, a fine soft-tipped sucker is helpful, but this should not be introduced into the vessel ends. An instrument that combines suction and irrigation is useful at this juncture (Evans et al 1983).

For end-to-side anastomosis the cutting of the side hole in the recipient artery is a difficult step that demands great care (Ikuta et al 1975). It should be placed to allow a relaxed lie for the approaching artery, with no kinking or tension. It is helpful to excise a small ellipse of appropriate size – not more than one-third of the artery's circumference, or it tends to open up in an hourglass shape that can be difficult to suture to. This may be inevitable when anastomosing a larger (end) to a smaller (side) artery, and the important measurement to balance is the length of cut vessel edge in the two openings, which should match as far as possible. Since the natural direction of flow from a side hole in an artery is at 90° to the line of the artery, the artery of the flap should be sutured to it at 90°, although it will take up the position that surrounding structures impose on it. The length of the suture line can be augmented by splitting one side of the approaching vessel and making a larger side opening to match, but there is usually no reason to do this.

Suturing should start at the far side in the direction from which the flap vessel is approaching, and should work round both sides in turn, leaving the more accessible nearside until last (Fig. 7.4). Particular care is needed to suture the back wall accurately, since later access to place additional sutures for control of leaks may be extremely difficult. If the pedicle does not easily reach the recipient vessels, vein grafts should be used. Preferably these would be planned from the start, so that adequate preparation can be made, but if difficulties arise during surgery, the decision to use vein grafts should be made easily and promptly, without wasting time trying to get by with a vessel repair under tension. For small vessels of digital artery size, the fine veins on the volar

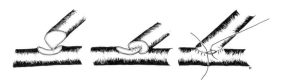

Fig. 7.4 Although it is possible to suture one side are then turn the vessels, it is often better to start with the far side and work round to the near side. The penultimate stitch can be left untied until the last stitch is placed.

aspect of the wrist are useful and readily available. Large veins from an arm or leg are needed for radial-artery sized vessels; if the arm is used, choice is limited by the need to preserve venous pathways that may be in use for flap drainage. The presence of valves dictates the direction of flow through a vein graft, which should be sutured in place at both ends before releasing the clamps. End-to-side anastomosis is preferable at the proximal end of an arterial vein graft, which should be inserted under slight tension, against the usual rules, because as soon as the graft fills with arterial blood it lengthens, and can become tortuous if it is not a snug fit. Godina (1986) advocated the use of arterial grafts for arterial reconstruction to avoid this problem, taking the thoracodorsal artery for this purpose (assuming that it is not already in use as the pedicle for a latissimus dorsi flap!).

If a vein graft tends to go into spasm before insertion it should be hydrostatically dilated by the forceful introduction of the patient's own blood, heparinized to prevent clotting.

On completion of both anastomoses the clamps should be removed first from the vein and then from the artery, taking the clamp off first on the side from which flow is coming. The anaesthetist should be warned that there may be some bleeding, and when there is muscle in the flap, that some ischaemic products will enter the circulation, sometimes with a transient fall in blood pressure. An antispasmodic of the calcium antagonist type can be used topically to inhibit arterial spasm: verapamil is useful from this point of view. The flap is inspected for the return of normal colour and capillary return (in the case of skin), bleeding from raw surfaces, and in the case of muscle, the return of contractility on electrical or physical stimulation. If the circulation fails to return, or if it returns then ceases again, the anastomoses should be checked for patency. The vessel is gently held with two pairs of vessel dilators close together at a point downstream from the anastomosis; the distal one is then moved apart from the other, squeezing blood out of the intervening segment. The proximal one is then released and rapid filling indicates patency of the anastomosis. This test should not be repeated in case damage to the vessel occurs.

At this stage the artery is the most likely culprit, since early venous occlusion usually leads only to protracted bleeding and venous engorgement initially, with progressive colour changes and finally circulatory failure occurring later, depending on the size of the vascular bed of the flap.

Finishing

Only when the surgeon is completely satisfied that the circulation is fully restored should the operation be completed. This is the time of greatest danger, because critical judgement may be compromised by fatigue and a feeling that the main part of the operation is over. Attention should be given to haemostasis of the undersurface and margins of the flap, any other deep structures are repaired, and the wound is closed without tension. Drains should be used readily, although if suction drainage is employed the tip of the drainage catheter must be kept well away from the vessel repairs. If closure of any part of the wound margin requires tension it is better to use a free skin graft as a temporary or permanent closure. A raw muscle or fascial flap should be sutured loosely in place with fine absorbable sutures, and covered immediately with a mesh graft, expanded little or not at all. This can be sutured, but not held with a tie-over pressure dressing. The anaesthetic should not be reversed nor the patient leave the theatre until the circulation of the flap is fully stabilized and the surgeon quite satisfied. Nail-biting in the recovery room is to be avoided.

Free flaps are generally best kept on view and only slightly elevated. Any evidence of haematoma beneath the flap is an indication for re-exploration and removal under theatre conditions, avoiding damage to the pedicle by blind suction or probing. A single bleeding vessel may be found, or less commonly, an anastomotic leak, but more often,

no active bleeding is demonstrated. If there is generalized oozing which fails to settle, it is important to check the venous repair, since occlusion can result in such an occurrence initially, especially in a large flap, associated with swelling and cyanosis which can be difficult to detect at first.

Arterial failure is a commoner occurrence, and can be recognized by loss of the healthy oxygenated pink colour and capillary return. In a small flap the pallor occurs quickly and is obvious, but when the vascular bed is large colour changes are more insidious, and what appears to be capillary return may merely be the displacement of stagnant blood which creeps back (Khoo & Bailey 1982, Jones et al 1983). Later a mottled appearance develops as patchy vascular dilatation occurs with complete stagnation, and this is a sign of established arterial occlusion. The diagnosis should be made well before this occurs, and demands regular inspection by a trained eye (still the most reliable monitor), backed up by whatever more sophisticated monitoring systems are available. The photoplethysmograph is reliable but requires experienced interpretation (Webster & Patterson 1976, Harrison et al 1983, Scheker et al 1985). Temperature monitoring is more simply interpreted by less-trained staff, who are instructed to report a given temperature drop (2° below surrounding skin is an acceptable watershed, but this can be misleading and needs to be confirmed by trained observation) (Acland 1981, Leonard et al 1982, Jones et al 1983, Lu et al 1984). Muscle stimulation is useful when the muscle surface is on view, and is easily interpreted, with a time lag of 1 hour before contractility dies away after vascular occlusion (Batchelor et al 1982, Davison et al 1986). Care must be taken to avoid too strong a current, which can cause vigorous contraction and disruption of muscle sutures. The laser Doppler (Jones 1985) is sophisticated and quite reliable, but expensive. The best policy is to combine obsessional trained observation with one or two ancillary methods which one is used to interpreting (Jones 1985).

Any hint of vascular failure should prompt early reexploration. It is wise to set this in motion at the first sign of trouble, since the inevitable delay gives time for spontaneous recovery, and avoids losing time if there really is a problem. Early intervention can restore the circulation if a late thrombus develops in artery or vein, and there is no reason to regret reexploration if it is found that all is well. Occasionally all that needs to be done is to remove a small haematoma from around the vessels, and on one occasion the induction of general anaesthesia was swiftly followed by flap recovery!

Most vascular problems arise within 24 hours, but they can occur later, and some level of observation should be maintained for up to 5 days.

REVISION OF FREE FLAPS

The aim is to conclude the surgery in one stage, but occasionally subsequent procedures are necessary, for the repair or release of tendons, or nerve or bone surgery. Flaps may need thinning, and liposuction may be of value, augmented if necessary by selected fat excision. Generally it is preferable not to disrupt the pedicle while doing this, but if it happens by accident there is not likely to be a problem unless the flap is excessively undermined, or its margins are incised too extensively.

This chapter has emphasized in some detail the problems and pitfalls attending free tissue transfer to the hand. No doubt there are many more ways to lose a free flap, but cultivation of the right frame of mind to anticipate and deal with problems can make this an infrequent occurrence.

REFERENCES

Acland R D 1981 Surface temperature measurement: another useful method for free flap monitoring. Plastic and Reconstructive Surgery 68: 19

Albertengo J G, Rodriguez A, Buncke H J, Hall E J 1981 A comparative study of flap survival rates in end-to-end and end-to-side microvascular anastomoses. Plastic and Reconstructive Surgery 67: 194

Awwad A M, White R J, Lowe G D O, Forbes C D 1983a The effect of blood viscosity on blood flow in the experimental saphenous flap model. British Journal of Plastic Surgery 36: 383

Awwad A M, White R J, Webster M H C, Vance J P 1983b The effect of temperature on blood flow in island and free skin flaps: an experimental study. British Journal of Plastic Surgery 36: 373

Batchelor A G, Kay S, Evans D M 1982 A simple and effective method of monitoring free muscle transfer: a preliminary report. British Journal of Plastic Surgery 35: 343

Biemer E 1977 Vein grafts in microvascular surgery. British Journal of Plastic Surgery 30: 197

Buchler U, Phelps D B, Winspur I, Boswick J A 1977 The irrigation jet: an aid to microvascular surgery. Journal of Hand Surgery 2: 24

Chow S P, Huang C D, Chan C W 1982 Microvascular anastomosis of arteries under tension. British Journal of Plastic Surgery 35: 82

Coleman J J, Jurkiewcz M J 1984 Methods of providing sensation to anaesthetic areas. Annals of Plastic Surgery 12: 177

Coleman S, Anson B J 1961 Arterial patterns in the hand based on the study of specimens. Surgery, Gynaecology and Obstetrics 113: 409

Daniel R K, Taylor G I 1973 Distant transfer of an island flap by microvascular arterial anastomosis: a clinical technique. Plastic and Reconstructive Surgery 52: 111

Daniel R K, Terzis J, Midgley R D 1976 Restoration of sensation to an anaesthetic hand by a free neurovascular flap from the foot. Plastic and Reconstructive Surgery 57: 275

Davison P M, Batchelor A G, Wilson G R, Sully L 1986 The muscle twitch monitor: a rapid unequivocal method of monitoring free muscle transfers. British Journal of Plastic Surgery 39: 356

Dolmans S, Guinbert J C, Baudet J 1979 The upper arm flap. Journal of Microsurgery 1: 162

Evans D M, Weightman B, Deane G 1983 A new suction irrigation device: uses in microsurgery and plastic surgery. British Journal of Plastic Surgery 36: 273

Foucher G, Hoang P, Citron N et al 1986 Joint reconstruction following trauma. Comparison of microsurgical transfer and conventional methods. A report of 61 cases. Journal of Hand Surgery, 11B: 388

Godina M 1979 Preferential use of end-to-side arterial anastomosis in free flap transfers. Plastic and Reconstructive Surgery 64: 673

Godina M 1986 Arterial autografts in microvascular surgery. Plastic and Reconstructive Surgery 78: 293

Godina M 1987 The tailored latissimus dorsi free flap. Plastic and Reconstructive Surgery 80: 304

Harashino T, Buncke H J 1975 Study of washout solutions for microvascular replantation and transplantation. Plastic and Reconstructive Surgery 50: 542

Harris G D, Finseth F, Buncke H J 1981 Posterior-wall-first microvascular anastomotic technique. British Journal of Plastic Surgery 34: 47

Harrison D M, Girling M, Mott G 1983 Methods of assessing the viability of free flap transfer during the postoperative period. Clinics in Plastic Surgery 10: 21

Ikuta Y, Watari S, Kawamura K et al 1975 Free flap transfer by end-to-side arterial anastomosis. British Journal of Plastic Surgery 28: 1

Jones B M, 1985 Predicting the fate of free tissue transfers. Annals of the Royal College of Surgeons 67: 63

Jones B M, Dunscombe P B, Greenhalgh R M 1983 Monitoring skin flaps by colour measurement. British Journal of Plastic Surgery 36: 88

Katsaros J, Schusterman M, Beppu M et al 1984 The lateral arm flap: anatomy and clinical applications. Annals of Plastic Surgery 12: 489

Khoo C T K, Bailey B N 1982 The behaviour of free muscle and musculocutaneous flaps after early loss of axial blood supply. British Journal of Plastic Surgery 35: 43

Leonard A G, Brennan M D, Colville J 1982 The use of continuous temperature monitoring in the postoperative management of microvascular cases. British Journal of Plastic Surgery 35: 337

Lu S Y, Chin S Y, Lin T, Chen M T 1984 Evaluation of survival in digital replantation with thermometric monitoring. Journal of Hand Surgery 9A: 804

McCraw J B, Furlow L T 1975 The dorsalis pedis arterialized flap. Plastic and Reconstructive Surgery 55: 177

McGregor I A, Jackson I T 1972 The groin flap. British Journal of Plastic Surgery 25: 3

Manktelow R T, Zucker R M, McKee N H 1984 Functioning free muscle transplantation. Journal of Hand Surgery 9A: 32

Mathes S J, Buchanan R T 1979 Tensor fascia lata neurosensory musculocutaneous free flaps. British Journal of Plastic Surgery 32: 184

May J W, Chait L A, Cohen B E, O'Brien 1977 Free neurovascular flap from the first web of the foot in hand reconstruction. Journal of Hand Surgery 2: 387

Morrison W A, O'Brien B M, MacLeod A M 1980 Thumb reconstruction with a free neurovascular wraparound flap from the big toe. Journal of Hand Surgery 5: 575

Nolan J, Jenkins R A, Kurihara K, Schulz R L 1985 The acute effects of cigarette smoke exposure on experimental skin flaps. Plastic and Reconstructive Surgery 75: 544

Rowsell A R, Godfrey A M, Richards M A 1986 The thinned latissimus dorsi free flap: a case report. British Journal of Plastic Surgery 39: 210

Scheker L R, Slattery P G, Firrell J C, Lister G D 1985 The value of the photoplethysmograph in monitoring skin closure in microsurgery. Journal of Reconstructive Microsurgery 2: 1

Smith P J 1982 The Y-shaped hypogastric groin flap. Hand 14: 263

Terzis J K, Sweet R C, Dykes R W, Williams H B 1978 Recovery of function in free muscle transplants using microvascular anastomoses. Journal of Hand Surgery 3: 37

Tobin G R, Shusterman M, Peterson G H et al 1981 The intramuscular neurovascular anatomy of the latissimus dorsi muscle flap: the basis for splitting the flap. Plastic and Reconstructive Surgery 67: 637

Upton J, Rogers C, Durham-Smith G, Swartz W M 1986 clinical applications of free temporoparietal flaps in hand reconstruction. Journal of Hand Surgery 11A : 475

Webster M H C, Patterson J 1976 the photo-electric plethysmograph as a monitor of microvascular anastomoses. British Journal of Plastic Surgery 29: 182

Wood M, Irons G B 1983 Upper extremity free skin flap: results and utility as compared with conventional distant pedicle skin flaps. Annals of Plastic Surgery 11: 523

The lateral arm free flap

INTRODUCTION

The lateral arm flap is a relatively new flap which came into prominence when first described by Song in 1982. Its use has also been reported by Matloub et al (1983) and Schusterman et al (1983). On casual consideration, it is a most unlikely candidate to emerge as a popular flap in the treatment of upper extremity skin loss. The questions which arise are, firstly, whether its vascular supply is as reliable as that of either the forearm flap or the latissimus dorsi flap, and secondly, whether the vessels are likely to be large enough for easy anastomosis. Also, it seems at first glance that there are two major factors which could preclude this procedure from routine use – the apparently limited amount of skin available and the likelihood of an ugly donor site. Usually these fears are expressed because of a lack of first-hand knowledge of the anatomy, and of experience in the various applications of the flap. In fact, the more one uses this flap, the more one gains the type of information which can expand the limits of its application.

For example, a surprisingly large area of skin can be taken without having to apply a skin graft to the donor site, especially in older patients. Even larger areas of skin loss can be covered by splitting the flap (see page 93). The rich blood supply of the flap and its constant anatomy also provide great comfort to the surgeon, who learns to raise it with easy wide-open access to the vascular pedicle. The most pleasant surprise, however, has been the low donor-site morbidity. In particular the cosmetic disability has been less than expected

and certainly compares favourably with that of other procedures.

The anatomical information presented in this chapter is based on 32 cadaver dissections (Katsaros et al 1984) and 132 clinical cases, of which 42 involved the repair of skin loss to the upper extremity.

ANATOMY

The longitudinal axis of the flap, identified by a line joining the acromion to the lateral epicondyle, indicates the surface marking of the flap's axial supply – the profunda brachii vessels (Fig. 8.1). These course alongside the humerus in the spiral groove and emerge at the deltoid insertion to extend beyond that into the substance of the lateral intermuscular septum (Fig. 8.2.). Beyond the deltoid insertion, the profunda brachii artery continues as the posterior radial collateral artery, after giving off major branches which accompany the radial nerve trunk anteriorly and which enter the triceps posteriorly. The posterior radial collateral

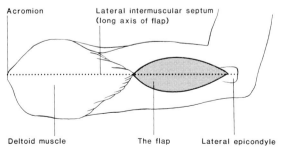

Fig. 8.1 Surface markings of the standard lateral arm flap.

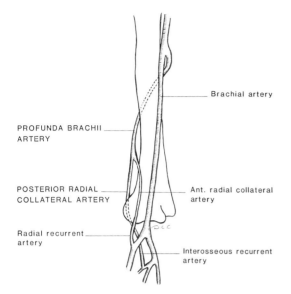

Fig. 8.2 Vascular anatomy of the upper arm, showing the arterial supply to the flap, the posterior radial collateral artery arising from the profunda brachii.

artery is therefore the major axial artery within the flap, giving off small muscular and cutaneous branches which radiate both anteriorly and posteriorly. Whilst most identifiable skin branches are seen distal to the deltoid insertion there is a constant proximal branch supplying the skin over the deltoid muscle. The largest cutaneous branch of this axial system is found just distal to this deltoid branch, and is up to 1 mm wide in adult male patients. The constancy of these two branches is an important factor in the 'split' flap modification discussed later.

Other distal cutaneous branches are small, but are nevertheless easily seen and are significant contributors to the vascularity of the distal portion of the flap. Two cutaneous nerves accompany the vessels through the territory of the flap. The posterior cutaneous nerve of the arm divides into three or four identifiable twigs which ramify into the skin of the overlying triceps. The posterior cutaneous nerve of the forearm passes through the lateral intermuscular septum, and accompanied by one of the anterior cutaneous branches of the artery, provides sensation to the skin over the brachioradialis and the lateral forearm. This nerve has a substantial diameter which ranges from 1 mm to 2 mm. In general, its thickness tends to be approximately 75% of that of the sural nerve.

The two veins in the pedicle tend to be 3 mm and 1 mm in diameter respectively, but often these meet to form a single trunk deep in the spiral groove. The calibre of the artery varies between 1 mm and 2.5 mm; it is more likely to be 1 mm in females, whilst diameters of 2 mm or more are seen only in athletic adult males. Most commonly, the profunda brachii is 1.5 mm in diameter and the length of the vascular pedicle is 7–8 cm.

The dimensions of skin which could be raised on the profunda brachii artery have yet to be determined. Latex injection studies in fresh specimens produce a cutaneous flare over the lateral arm which is approximately 10 cm × 10 cm in area. In theory, a tube of skin of the entire brachium extending to the mid-forearm could be taken. This has never been proven clinically.

Anatomical variations

In all the cadaver studies (Katsaros et al 1984) and all the clinical cases there was no absence of the profunda or posterior radial collateral vessels. In six instances there was duplication of the arterial system, with corresponding reduction of the calibre of vessels. There has been minimal variation in the distribution of cutaneous nerves.

OPERATIVE TECHNIQUE FOR RAISING THE FLAP

Under ideal circumstances the patient is placed in the supine position under general anaesthesia, although regional anaesthesia is suitable. Foam wedges are placed under the shoulder and hip to produce an elevation of approximately 30°. This brings the lateral arm area into a suitable orientation so that the arm lies on the chest wall in the midaxillary line. Owing to this inclination there is no tendency for the arm to fall backwards below the level of the costal cartilages, and the surgeon can work comfortably without stooping. The area is shaved, prepared and draped from the clavicle to the wrist.

The longitudinal axis of the flap is marked from the acromion to the lateral epicondyle. The surface marking of the profunda brachii artery is identified on this line near the deltoid insertion.

The area of skin to be taken is then outlined, taking into account the fact that the flap is supplied by branches which arise sequentially between the deltoid insertion and the lateral epicondyle. The line drawn between these should be in the middle of any skin flap raised, irrespective of its size. If this is not strictly observed when raising small flaps, there is a risk that the axial blood supply may be excluded from the skin paddle. Usually the skin flap is marked out as an ellipse (Fig. 8.1), but any desired shape is feasible.

To create ideal operating conditions a tourniquet is then applied. This may be a paediatric inflatable type, or of the Esmarch variety. A thin rubber (Martin's) bandage is preferred because it can be applied high up near the axilla without intruding on the operative field.

First the arm is exsanguinated by winding the bandage from the wrist towards the axilla, and then arterial occlusion is achieved with three revolutions of the bandage as near to the axilla as possible. The skin incisions are then made through to muscle both anteriorly (brachialis, brachioradialis, extensor carpi radialis longus and brevis) and posteriorly (triceps). The key to finding the vessels and raising the flap quickly is to begin posteriorly and proceed deep to the investing fascia of triceps. Small cutaneous branches are seen glistening through fascia and these are followed to their origin from the profunda – posterior radial collateral system. Muscle branches are divided until the axial system coursing within the lateral intermuscular septum is displayed. The septum is divided near its attachment to the humerus between the deltoid insertion and the lateral epicondyle.

The anterior subfascial dissection is then directed in the same way towards the axial vessels, until the cut edge of the intermuscular septum is encountered. At this point the anterior and posterior dissections come into continuity.

The flap distal to the lateral epicondyle is then raised above the fascia, preserving the ligamentous fibres of the extensor mass origin. Just proximal to the lateral epicondyle, where the extensors consist of red fleshy fibres, the fascia is incised thus joining the distal and proximal parts of the dissection. Proceeding in a distal-to-proximal direction, muscle branches are divided from the axial system

until the profunda artery is encountered in the spiral groove. At this point only the vessels and cutaneous nerves should be preserved, which implies that all fascial connections between the flap and nearby muscles should be severed. The surgeon can become 'lost' at this point unless the course of the profunda vessels in the spiral groove is followed closely, without retaining any fascial covering. To gain greater length in the pedicle, the fascial roof of the spiral groove is incised at the junction of triceps and deltoid muscles. This is facilitated by using a small self-retaining retractor which helps to separate these muscles and display the vessels more clearly. The radial nerve can then be identified in a deeper plane lying close to bone. The profunda artery and comitantes may be divided at the appropriate place, along with the cutaneous nerves which can easily be distinguished from the main trunk of the radial nerve. After removal of the tourniquet, haemostasis is achieved before wound closure is performed. Defects 6 cm wide (10 cm wide in elderly patients) can be closed without difficulty.

RATIONALE FOR USING THE FLAP

In discussing the alternatives for vascularized skin cover in the hand, this flap should be compared with the most commonly used procedure – the radial forearm flap, used either as a distally based island flap or a free flap from the opposite forearm. In the face of overwhelming proof that the forearm flap is a reliable thin flap with large calibre vessels and a long pedicle, what attractions does the lateral arm flap have by comparison? The question may also be asked whether it should be preferred under any circumstances. There are three main reasons to justify such a choice.

1. The individual surgeon's preference
2. The lateral arm donor site can be closed directly without a skin graft
3. The major arteries of the hand are preserved.

In direct comparison the forearm donor site invariably requires a skin graft for closure. It is also acknowledged that surgeons frequently experience difficulty in achieving complete skin-graft take over the flexor carpi radialis tendon, and this may result in delayed healing.

The lateral arm flap can be raised on the same extremity which has sustained the hand injury, even though the transverse carpal arteries may be damaged. It would not be wise to raise a radial forearm flap under the same circumstances for fear of devascularizing the digits. Generally, the radial forearm flap vessels are of greater calibre than those of the lateral arm, but with the level of microsurgical expertise available in most hand units the anastomoses do not present any particular problem.

The radial forearm pedicle is longer than the lateral arm pedicle, which may be 8 cm long in the adult. For most clinical situations, however, 8 cm is an adequate length and compares favourably with other commonly used skin flaps such as groin and scapular flaps.

With regard to the reliability of the blood supply, experience suggests that the profunda brachii artery is as constant as the radial artery. Duplication and reduction in artery calibre, however, is more likely to occur with the profunda brachii artery. It is acknowledged that the forearm flap is thinner than the lateral arm flap, but both flaps are fat and unattractive in obese individuals. When a lateral arm flap is taken distal to the deltoid insertion and extends on to the forearm, the tissue may be acceptably thin (Figs 8.3B,C). When a longer flap extending proximally over the deltoid is taken, the lateral arm flap is likely to be bulky and require later revision.

In other respects such as operative access, ease of raising the flap and surface area of the skin, the flaps are comparable. Initially it was felt that the lateral arm flap was not appropriate for use in young women and children, because of the po-

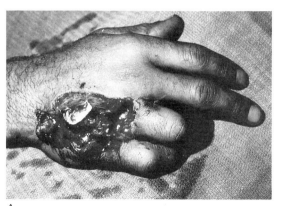

A

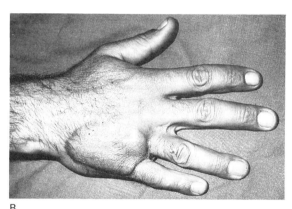

B

C

Fig. 8.3 Case No.1. **A** Compound intra-articular fractures of the right fourth and fifth rays in a 26-year-old farmhand who fell from his motorcycle. **B** Appearance of dorsum of hand 1 year after injury. **C** Right hand held in flexion 1 year later.

tential for unsightly scarring. However, this has not been found to be the case and surprisingly good cosmetic results are seen in these two groups.

CONVENTIONAL LATERAL ARM FLAP

Case report

A 26-year-old farm hand was thrown from his motorcycle in a collision with a motorcar. The force of the impact was borne by the dorsum of the hand as he struck the ground. Clinical and radiological assessment indicated compound intra-articular fractures of the fourth and fifth meta-carpals (Fig. 8.3A). Skin loss measured 6 cm × 8 cm. Under general anaesthesia the wounds were debrided and the metacarpals realigned with Kirschner pins. A lateral arm flap taken from the same limb was used to cover the defect at the primary operation. The profunda brachii artery was anastomosed to the ulnar artery in an end-to-side fashion. The flap vein was anastomosed to a surface vein of the forearm. The patient was discharged from hospital 7 days later and physical rehabilitation commenced. Eighteen months after the injury he was employed as the driver of grading machinery without experiencing signifi-cant disability. His range of motion at the meta-carpophalangeal joints was reduced by 30° but was painfree. No surgical revision was necessary (Figs 8.3B,C).

MODIFICATIONS OF THE FLAP

'Split' flap

This technique has been developed to cater for large areas of skin loss on the hand. It has resulted in the ability to cover defects up to 14 cm wide and yet still achieve direct closure of the donor defect. As mentioned above, the width of the lateral arm flap which can be taken comfortably is 6 cm. In adults it is common to achieve a flap width of 7 cm and in elderly patients up to 10 cm wide. The length which may be achieved is 35 cm in some adults. The planning and execution of a split flap to cover a hand defect measuring 15 cm × 14 cm is as follows: in the first step, a lateral arm

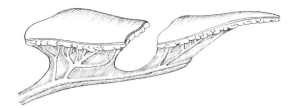
Fig. 8.4 The lateral arm flap split into two islands.

flap 30 cm long and 7 cm wide is raised from the deltoid area down to the forearm. Near the midpoint, the skin and subcutaneous fat are di-vided between two identifiable cutaneous arterial branches. The axial vascular system is preserved, thus splitting the flap into two islands which are both vascularized by the profunda brachii pos-terior collateral radial system (Fig. 8.4). The two islands of skin can then be rotated to lie side by side, so that the width of the flap is 14 cm (7+7) and its length is 15 cm. The donor site may then be closed directly as for small flaps, thereby mini-mizing the cosmetic deformity. The rationale for this modification is that a long scar is more accept-able than a skin graft on the lateral arm (Fig. 8.5).

Kinking of the vascular pedicle between the two segments has not been a problem: in fact, more difficulty is encountered if the splitting manoeuvre is tentative. A bold dissection which fashions true island flaps allows a comfortable rotation of the pedicle through 180° without kinking.

Case report

A 19-year-old boy sustained a severe wound to the

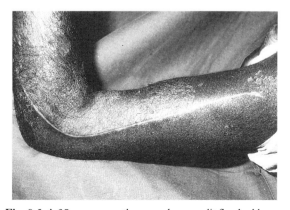
Fig. 8.5 A 35 cm scar on the arm where a split flap had been taken to resurface the dorsum of the hand.

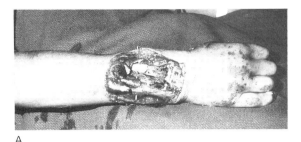
A

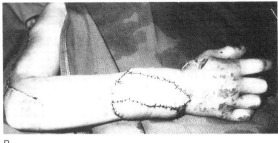
B

Fig. 8.6 Case No.2. **A** Dorsum of the right wrist in a 9-year-old boy involved in a motorcar accident. **B** Postoperative appearance, showing the two segments of the split flap covering the wrist defect. The donor site has been closed directly.

dorsum of the right hand in a motorcar accident, which resulted in loss of skin, subcutaneous tissue and extensor tendons. The distal radius, wrist joint and intercarpal joints were exposed. He was taken to the operating theatre on the day of injury and after thorough debridement and irrigation, a lateral arm flap measuring 20 cm × 4 cm was raised on the same arm. This was split into two segments and used to cover the defect, which measured 10 cm × 8 cm. The wound healed primarily, but he later developed degenerative changes in the carpus. The immediate pre- and postoperative appearance of the hand is shown in Figs 8.6A & B.

NEUROSENSORY FLAP

Owing to the fact that the posterior cutaneous nerve of the arm provides sensation to the lateral arm area, the flap has neurosensory potential. The likelihood of achieving high quality discriminatory sensibility is small, however, and at best protective sensation may be the end result. For the palmar aspect of the hand or digits, it is unlikely to surpass the quality of a pulp or web-space free-tissue transfer from the foot.

As outlined in the anatomical discussion, the posterior cutaneous nerve of the forearm courses with the vessels and passes over the extensor muscles into the forearm. It is therefore a source of vascularized nerve graft with a diameter similar to that of a digital nerve. If the posterior cutaneous nerve does not overlie the digital nerve defect, it may not be possible to retain the nerve's vascular connections, in which case it may be used as a conventional free nerve graft.

Case report

An 18-year-old woman was involved in a motorcar accident in which her right hand sustained full-thickness skin loss on the palm. The abrasion injury had resulted in loss of the radial digital nerve of the index finger and exposure of the flexor tendons to the same digit. Three days after the initial debridement on the day of injury, a lateral arm flap measuring 8 cm × 5 cm was raised to cover the right palmar defect. The lateral cutaneous nerve of the forearm was taken as a free non-vascularized graft to bridge a 6 cm defect in the radial digital nerve to the index. The nerve to the flap, the posterior cutaneous nerve of the forearm, was sutured to a branch of the radial sensory nerve on the dorsum of the hand, where full-thickness skin abrasion had also occurred. This small area measuring 3 cm × 3 cm was covered with a split-thickness skin graft. Three Z-plasties were placed along the radial suture line, and in particular into the first web space.

Primary skin healing occurred with minimal pin-cushioning of the flap. Scar contracture did not develop in the web space and full range of motion of all joints was achieved. Twelve months after repair the two-point discrimination on the radial side of the index finger measured 8 mm. Protective sensation was achieved in the skin flap, which did not require revision. This case is illustrated in Figs 8.7A–D.

FASCIAL FLAP

In obese individuals, or when an ultra-thin flap is required, fascia only may be used. Split-thickness

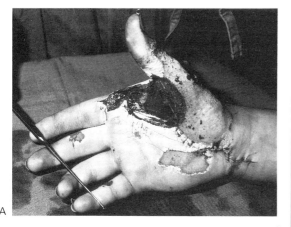

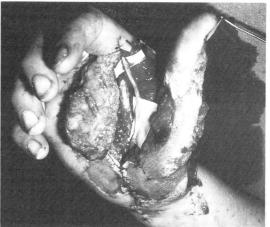

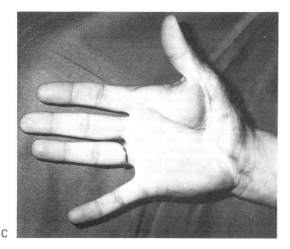

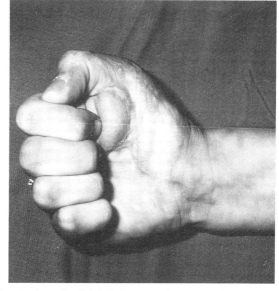

Fig. 8.7 Case No.3. **A** The palmar defect in an 18-year-old girl, showing loss of radial digital nerve and exposure of the flexor tendons. **B** The posterior cutaneous nerve of the forearm has been grafted into the digital nerve defect as a non-vascularized graft. **C** Digital extension at 12 months, with two-point discrimination of 8 mm in right index. **D** Digital flexion preserved.

skin graft is applied to the revascularized fat and fascia to achieve closure of large or small defects of the hand. This technique is most appropriate for obese patients, in whom a flap from any site would be excessively bulky. Although this type of reconstruction has been performed elsewhere on the body (forehead, dorsum of foot), it has not been used in the treatment of hand injuries. For this reason an example of the same technique used in a case of a foot injury is shown. It should be noted that the fascia does not appear to sustain a skin

graft beyond the vascular territory outlined by latex or fluorescein injection studies. This has been observed consistently in clinical cases. It is therefore implied that fascia taken distal to the lateral epicondyle is unlikely to nourish a skin graft. In fact, it has been noted that skin grafts in general do not take well when applied to the fascial flap initially. In most cases a second skin-grafting procedure has been performed when healthy granulations appear, approximately 1 week later. The reason for this is not clear, but it

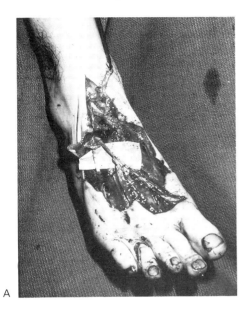

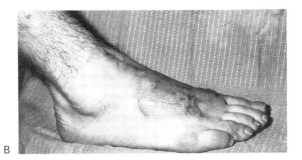

Fig. 8.8 Case No 4. **A** Foot injury in a 38-year-old man. **B** Appearance of the foot 6 months after repair with a fascial flap and skin graft. Note the absence of contour deformity.

may be related to the lack of lymphatic drainage from the flap.

Case report

This case of a foot injury illustrates this modification, which can be applied in a similar fashion to injuries of the upper extremity.

A 38-year-old factory worker sustained a degloving injury to the right foot, which was caught in a conveyor belt. Extensor tendons, intertarsal joints and metatarsal shafts were exposed over an area measuring 12 cm × 14 cm. After debridement, the repaired structures were covered by a fascial lateral arm flap, which in turn was covered with a split-skin graft. Initially there was 50% patchy skin-graft take. Ten days later a second skin-grafting procedure was necessary to achieve final healing. The patient was discharged from hospital 3 weeks after the injury and primary fascial flap cover. Figures 8.8A & B illustrate the features of this case.

VASCULARIZED TENDON GRAFT

Vascularized triceps tendon may be taken with the skin flap by preserving muscular arteries which branch off posteriorly, as mentioned above. Usually it is necessary to take approximately 1 cm

thickness of triceps with an appropriate strip of triceps tendon, which is flat and ribbon-like. It is possible to remove approximately 15 cm × 1.5 cm of tendon without significantly affecting triceps function. Closure of the secondary defect is performed in the usual way by closing the skin directly over muscle. This technique has been used to bridge extensor tendon defects, but has not been tried on the flexor side of the hand. In five patients the results have been disappointing, due to severe adhesions which can partly be attributed to the severity of the injury. In fact the triceps tendon is not a good substitute for hand extensors, and it may be more appropriate to consider conventional grafting at a later stage after a skin flap has been applied. Vascularized triceps tendon has been used more successfully in the segmental replacement of larger tendons such as the tendo Achilles.

Case report

A 21-year-old male student sustained skin and extensor tendon loss on the dorsum of the right hand in a motorcar accident. The patient's right arm was outside the vehicle at the time of impact, which resulted in abrasion of all soft tissues down to the metacarpal shafts (Fig. 8.9A). Under general anaesthetic on the day of injury, a split lateral arm flap, taken with vascularized triceps tendon,

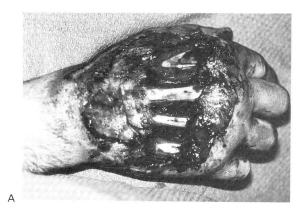

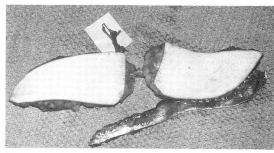

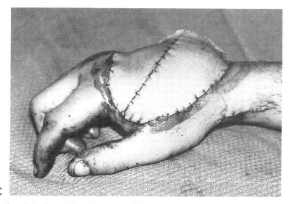

Fig. 8.9 Case No. 5. **A** Injury to the right hand in a 21-year-old male. **B** A split flap is taken, with vascularized triceps tendon. **C** Postoperative appearance following tendon reconstruction and skin cover.

was used to reconstruct the long extensor tendons and provide skin cover (Figs 8.9B,C). Satisfactory wound healing occurred, but extensor tendon function remained poor. A tenolysis procedure was performed without significant improvement. The severity of the original injury was felt to be the main reason for widespread fibrosis around the extensor tendons.

OSTEOCUTANEOUS FLAP

A strut of humerus may be incorporated in the flap by preserving muscular and periosteal branches adjacent to the attachment of the lateral intermuscular septum. A cuff of muscle 1 cm wide is taken with the flap on either side of the septum. A length of supracondylar ridge 10 cm long and up to 1.5 cm wide can be taken between the lateral epicondyle and the deltoid insertion. The radial nerve trunk must be identified and protected

when the bone is cut using an oscillating micro saw (Fig. 8.10). The graft is mainly cortical bone, and is not vascularized by large nutrient vessels at this site. Small vessels are sometimes seen entering bone through small foramina. This is most useful in reconstructing metacarpal loss, but

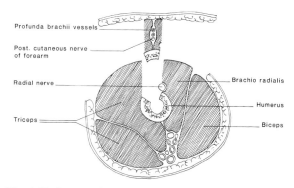

Fig. 8.10 Cross-section of arm showing the configuration of the osteocutaneous flap. Approximately one-sixth of the circumference of the humerus can be taken safely.

defects of the proximal phalanx of the thumb and the radius have also been treated successfully by this method. The diameter of the humerus is larger than that of the radius and hence fracture has not been a problem, as is the case with the radial forearm osteocutaneous flap.

Case report

A 32-year-old industrial worker was referred for reconstruction of the right third metacarpal 2 months after a severe punch-press injury. He presented with an external fixator which maintained length in the shattered metacarpal. There was a 4 cm segmental loss in the midshaft area. A lateral arm osteocutaneous flap, incorporating 4 cm of the supracondylar ridge of the humerus, was transferred in an elective operation to reconstruct

the defect. The bone graft was dowelled at either end, such that metal fixation was unnecessary. Satisfactory hand function was achieved at 3 months, permitting his return to work. Pre- and postoperative X-rays are shown in Figs 8.11A & B.

THE MINI FLAP

The most agonizing problem to deal with in terms of making a decision is the case of the small compound defect. With extensive injuries there is less hesitation in applying a microsurgical solution, compared with the small defect where the surgeon may be tempted to try closure with local tissues or a pedical flap. Under these circumstances local flap procedures must be executed perfectly,

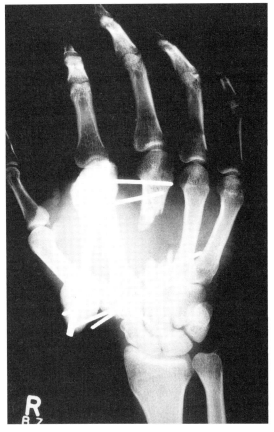
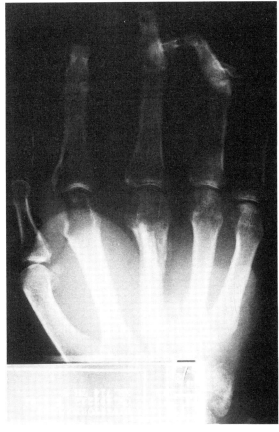

A   B

Fig. 8.11 Case No.6 **A** Radiograph of metacarpal loss in a 32-year-old punch-press operator. **B** Postoperative appearance showing reconstruction with vascularized humerus osteocutaneous flap.

to avoid further skin loss through tension. If it is recognized that a local flap repair may be hazardous, the lateral arm flap can be considered as a realistic alternative to the pedicled cross-arm or abdominal flap repair. Flaps which are a little more than the size of a postage stamp may be raised near the lateral epicondyle and used to close compound defects of the digits. This method is especially useful for defects of the thumb. To counter criticism that the procedure takes 3–4 hours, it can be argued that the patient is saved further hospitalization, or additional surgery and morbidity associated with pedicled flaps.

Case report

A 55-year-old farmer sustained a compound fracture of the proximal phalanx of the right thumb, which had been caught in a winching machine (Fig. 8.12A). On the day of injury a debridement

was performed under general anaesthesia. A bone graft from the subcutaneous border of the right ulna was taken to bridge a 2 cm long defect in the proximal phalanx. Local skin was used to cover the dorsum of the digit, but it was noted that closure was achieved with tension on the local skin flaps. During the next 7 days the extent of skin flap necrosis became evident (Fig. 8.12B). Eight days after injury, a small lateral arm skin flap measuring 4 cm × 2 cm was used to cover the extensor tendon and bone graft of the thumb. The lateral arm flap vessels were anastomosed end-to-side to the radial artery in the anatomical snuffbox. Postoperatively, primary skin healing occurred and the bone graft united solidly (Figs 8.12C,D). Metacarpophalangeal and interphalangeal joint range of motion were reduced by 20%. He returned to work on the farm 3 months after injury and did not require revision of the skin flap.

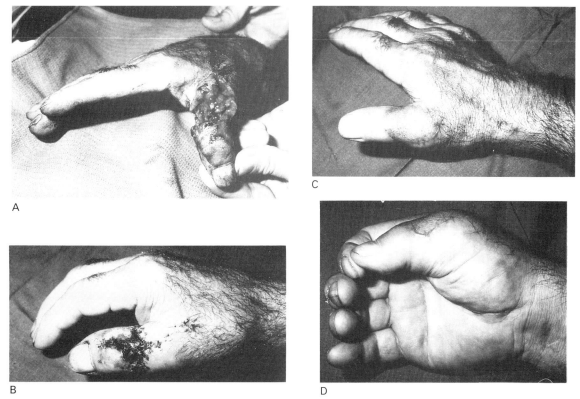

Fig. 8.12 Case No. 7 **A** Skin and bone loss in the thumb of a 55-year-old farmer. **B** Necrosis of local skin flaps after bone and tendon graft. **C** Appearance of thumb 6 months after lateral arm flap repair. **D** Lateral view showing thinness of the flap.

COMPLICATIONS

Some of the pitfalls of this procedure have been alluded to in the preceding text. In summary they may be categorized as complications related to the donor site, or as complications of the flap itself.

Donor site

Nerve compression has been the commonest and the most serious problem, occurring in four out of 132 patients (3%). This has been related to the use of the tourniquet in three cases, where all three major nerves of the limb were affected but recovered completely within 4 weeks. In the fourth patient a transient posterior interosseous palsy occurred because a tight closure was performed over the long extensors of the wrist. It was necessary to decompress the nerve and apply a skin graft 2 days after the initial operation. This could have been avoided by narrowing the flap distal to the lateral epicondyle, or by planning the flap at a more proximal site in the upper arm. Alternatively a skin graft could have been used after recognizing that the closure would be tight.

When using a tourniquet, care should be taken to avoid high compression in the arm by using a calibrated paediatric inflatable cuff, or by applying a maximum of three revolutions when using an Esmarch-type tourniquet. The latter method requires practice and experience to achieve just enough compression to occlude arterial inflow.

Delayed wound healing

Wounds of the lateral arm may be slow to heal after direct closure, for a variety of reasons. Associated factors may be wound infection at the site of subcutaneous suture where catgut has been used. Skin sutures which are removed too early may also contribute to wound dehiscence over the lateral epicondyle, where skin closure is often tightest. Wound seroma requiring drainage may occur if suction drains are removed prematurely.

Based on clinical experience, the following recommendations are made to minimize wound healing problems:

1. Avoid absorbable subcuticular sutures which may lead to localized infection
2. Use monofilament synthetic suture
3. Reduce elbow motion in the first week
4. Maintain suction drainage for 7 days
5. Remove skin sutures after 3 weeks.

Cosmetic deformity

In most cases of hand injury it is possible to raise the lateral arm flap on the same limb. This confines the scars to one extremity and is preferable to the disfigurement of another area, such as the opposite forearm.

The most unsightly lateral arm defect is produced when skin grafting is necessary. Efforts to minimize cosmetic deformity, therefore, are aimed towards achieving a direct closure which is tension-free. The application of the split flap and fascial flap techniques help to reduce the breadth of donor-site defects. In general, wound closure with tension is more likely to produce an unsightly scar. Widened hypertrophic scars are seen more commonly in younger patients where direct closure has been tight. These undesirable features are more evident over the lateral epicondyle, where excessive motion during elbow flexion may be a contributing factor. Overall, the technique of direct skin closure has proved satisfactory, with skin grafting being necessary in only 3% of patients. A comparison of representative donor sites is shown in Figs 8.13, 8.14 and 8.15.

Injury to the radial nerve

Direct injury to the radial nerve in raising the flap

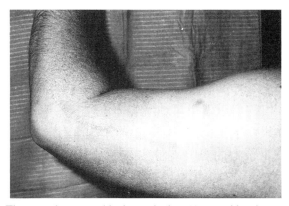

Fig. 8.13 An acceptable donor site in a 40-year-old male.

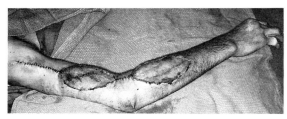

Fig. 8.14 Postoperative appearance in a man in whom a 35 cm x 8 cm flap was taken. Skin grafting was necessary both above and below the lateral epicondyle.

has not occurred, even though this structure is at risk of accidental damage on every occasion. It could be argued that such a complication should never occur, but precautions must be taken to avoid this disastrous complication, including:

1. Familiarity with the anatomy
2. Use of the tourniquet to achieve a bloodless operating field when possible
3. Judicious use of bipolar diathermy near the radial nerve
4. Taking extra care when raising the osteocutaneous flap
5. Practice in raising the flap in the anatomy laboratory.

PROBLEMS RELATED TO THE FLAP

Anatomical variations

The most frequently observed anomaly is duplication of the profunda artery. This does not create any difficulty in males, where each artery may be 1 mm in diameter, but in females the vessel dia-

meter tends to be less, and a duplicated artery of 0.75 mm or less may create technical anastomotic difficulties. If the vascular pedicle is traced proximally high up in the spiral groove, duplicated arteries often combine to a common trunk. Taking the artery proximal to this point would eliminate a problem under these circumstances.

Cosmetic appearance of the flap

In obese individuals this flap is always fat, especially in its proximal part which overlies the deltoid muscle. It is more difficult to achieve a satisfactory wound closure on the dorsum of palm of the hand in these patients. There is very little scope for aesthetic contouring of such a flap, which remains unattractive until it is revised (Figs 8.16A,B). A fascial flap covered with skin

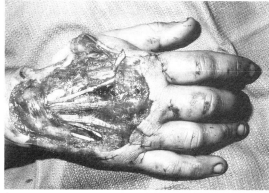

A

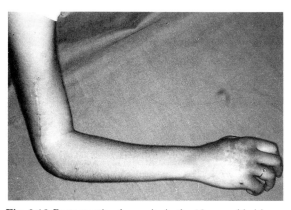

Fig. 8.15 Postoperative donor site in the 18-year-old girl presented in Case No. 3.

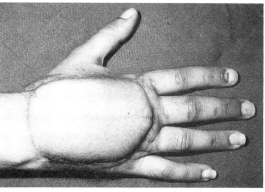

B

Fig. 8.16 A Appearance of hand injury in overweight female worker. **B** Appearance of fat lateral arm flap. A fascial flap would have given a better result.

graft would offer a superior result. On the other hand, a fat flap would be justified in cases of severe injury if the defect could be covered expeditiously, as this would offset the disadvantage of having to undertake a later thinning procedure.

The failing flap

On several occasions the failing flap has been salvaged after early postoperative thrombosis. It is easy to recognize arterial thrombosis, when the flap is typically pale and has lost turgor. Venous thrombosis, however, is not always associated with progressive cyanosis, as seen with the groin flap which finally assumes a blue-black colour. On three occasions when the flap was lost, venous thrombosis occurred first and was followed by arterial thrombosis before blue-black congestion occurred. A 'capillary refill' sign could be elicited after these thrombotic events and the flap was erroneously thought to be viable. In fact, on palpating the flap the refill sign indicated nothing more than a stagnant circulation where blood could neither enter nor leave the flap. On cursory inspection the flap appeared slightly congested, but generally pink. Close examination after removal of all bandages revealed early cyanosis at the edges of the flap.

As stated above, this clinical picture is seen because arterial thrombosis occurs soon after venous thrombosis is established. Without continued arterial input, dark-blue congestion does not occur and the stagnant blood in the flap appears mainly pink. This phenomenon has not been observed with such consistency when other flaps have been used, and no explanation springs to mind easily. Hence the message of caution is that one must be aware of the 'stagnant' lateral arm flap in which a 'normal' capillary refill test may be observed. Careful clinical monitoring is therefore advisable if flap-monitoring equipment is not available.

REFERENCES

Katsaros J, Schusterman M, Beppu M et al 1984 The lateral upper arm flap: anatomy and clinical applications. Annals of Plastic Surgery 12: 489

Matloub H S et al 1983 The lateral arm flap. A neurosensory free flap. In: Williams H B (ed) Transactions of the VIII International Congress of Plastic Surgery. Montreal, IPRS p. 125

Schusterman M, Beppu M, Banis J C 1983 The lateral arm flap, an experimental and clinical study. In: Williams H B (ed) Transactions of the VIII International Congress of Plastic Surgery. Montreal, IPRS, p. 132

Song R Y 1982 One-stage reconstructions. Clinics in Plastic Surgery 9: 1

The temporoparietal free flap

INTRODUCTION

Soft-tissue coverage with thin supple tissue in difficult regions along digits, within web spaces, the palm of the hand, and even the forearm has always been challenging for the hand surgeon. The introduction of the operating microscope has brought about a tremendous change in the approach to these reconstructive problems, and the temporoparietal fascia has emerged as a new, very versatile, donor site for localized problems in these difficult regions.

As a pedicle flap, this fascia has been used for the ear (Fox & Edgerton 1976), forehead (Byrd 1980), eyebrow, eyelid (Monks 1898, Byrd 1980) and temporomandibular joint reconstructions (Al-Kayat & Bramley 1979). As a free tissue transfer it was first used to cover chronic indolent wounds of the distal tibia and foot (Smith 1980, Brent et al 1985, Upton et al 1986), as a carrier for contralateral scalp transfers (Harii et al 1974), and to resurface total ear constructions (Brent & Byrd 1983). More recently, many applications within the hand and upper extremity have been presented (Upton 1985). Although other free fascial donor sites have been described in regions such as the calf (Walton & Bunkis 1984) and the lateral thigh (Song et al 1984), the parietotemporal donor region is still more practical, predictable and readily used for many upper extremity problems.

CLINICAL ANATOMY

The temporoparietal fascia represents the cephalic extension of the superficial musculoaponeurotic system (SMAS) which supports the muscles of facial expression (Mitz & Peyronie 1976, Couly et al 1985). It lies between the scalp and the fascia of the temporalis muscle and is continuous with the frontalis and occipitalis muscles. In the temporal

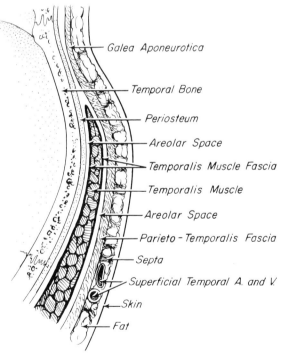

Fig. 9.1 A coronal section at the level of the temporal fossa demonstrates the relationship of the parietotemporal fascia to the overlying scalp and the underlying temporalis muscle. Note the fibrous septa which connect the external surface of the fascia and the dermis of the overlying scalp. A smooth areolar plane exists between the undersurface of the temporoparietal fascia and the fascia of the temporalis muscle. The superficial temporal artery and vein(s) always lie external to the fascia.

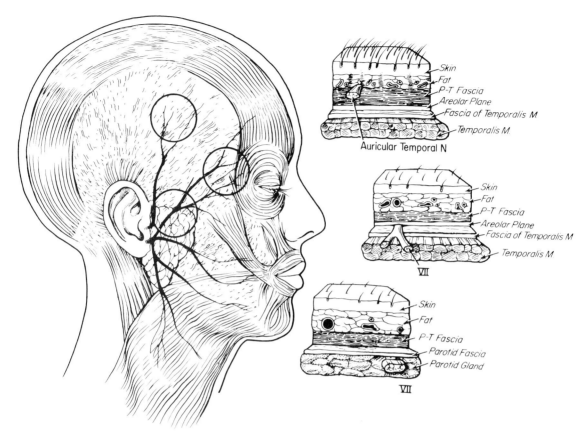

Fig. 9.2 The anatomical relationship of the nerves to this fascial layer are demonstrated. The sensory auriculotemporal nerve is the only nerve which lies *above* the fascia and the motor facial (VIIth) nerve is located *deep* to the fascia. The frontal and orbital branches of the VIIth nerve are vulnerable along the zygoma lateral to and above the orbital rim. (Inset right: below the level of the external auditory meatus the facial nerve lies deep within the parotid gland.)

region, separate longitudinal muscle fibres may be oriented along the long axis of this fascia which are not part of the frontalis or occipitalis muscle groups. Above the crest of the temporal fossa this layer becomes quite adherent to the scalp, and continues as the galea aponeurotica (Fig. 9.1). Fascial thickness in the midtemporal region varies tremendously with age, with measurements ranging from 2.0 mm to 4.3 mm. Cadaver and surgical dissections have shown this tissue to be consistently thin in the frontal region. At the end of a long surgical procedure, thickness may increase dramatically due to oedema. Thick, fibrous septa connect the external surface of the fascia to the dermis of the overlying scalp. As one progresses cephalad, the distance traversed by these connections decreases to the point where the fascia is almost adherent to the dermal layer

of scalp above the crest of the temporal fossa (Fig. 9.1). In contrast to its external surface, the internal side of this fascia has a smooth areolar surface, which creates a gliding plane between it and the fascia of the temporalis muscle. These anatomic characteristics make this tissue an ideal bed for gliding structures such as tendons.

Important nerves are always deep to the fascia and arteries are always superficial to it. The only nerve external to the parietotemporal fascia is the auriculotemporal nerve to the scalp. This sensory nerve courses anterior to the external auditory meatus and extends directly toward the dome of the calvarium, and does not necessarily follow vascular arborizations. It may routinely be sacrificed with the flap, particularly if scalp or hair-bearing tissue is to be included. Branches of the facial (VIIth) motor nerve are always found deep to the fascia. In the preauricular regions, the frontal and zygomatic branches are located well within the superficial lobe of the parotid gland and are not easily traumatized. Directly over or superior to the zygomatic process of the temporal bone, these arborizations become very superficial and are consistently located within the areolar plane beneath the temporoparietal fascia. Between two and four arborizations are usually found within 2.5–3.0 cm of the lateral canthus of the eye, a region where the nerve is most vulnerable to injury (Pitanguy & Silveira 1966). Dissection within this region should be avoided if possible (Fig. 9.2).

The axial vessels of this flap are the superficial temporal artery (STA) and vein(s) (STV), which are always found external to the temporoparietal fascia. Internal arterial diameter is large, measuring 1.8–2.5 mm at the level of the external auditory meatus. The accompanying vein is of much larger calibre – 2.1–3.5 mm – but its location may vary. In approximately 80% of the author's dissections it has been found within 1 cm of the artery, usually in an anterior location. In 20% of our dissections and clinical cases, it has been found either directly above (external) or posterior to the superficial temporal artery. Although a vein has always been present, the artery may be either unsuitable, hypoplastic, or of insufficient size for microanastomoses. A number of conditions which demonstrate abnormal and unpredictable vascular size and/or location include many craniofacial anomalies, particularly hemifacial microsomia, Romberg's disease (unilateral hemifacial atrophy), bilateral facial lipodystrophy, and congenital absence of the scalp and/or skull (cutis aplasia congenita). In severe forms of all of these conditions the fascia is usually insufficient for a free tissue transfer, but may be utilized locally as a pedicle flap. In addition, patients who have had previous temporomandibular joint surgery, corrective mandibular osteotomies or coronal scalp dissections, neurological or otherwise, may demonstrate a significant amount of scarring around these vessels. Marked distortion of both superficial temporal artery and vein have also been noted following altered growth secondary to childhood radiation for both benign and malignant diseases.

The subcutaneous depth of the superficial temporal artery and vein is important. In the parotid region these vessels lie within the upper portions of the gland but above the tragus of the ear; they are consistently found in a generous subcutaneous fat plane. At the crest of the temporal fossa, the fascia with its abundant anastomotic network is almost intradermal. This is the same region in which the fascia is closely adherent to the dermis of the scalp, where dissection of the fascia may be difficult, particularly in the region of the frontalis muscle (Fig. 9.3, heavily stippled area).

Five major branching patterns of the superficial temporal artery have been described, both recently and in the past (Eustathiasos 1932, Salmon 1936, Ricbourg et al 1975, Stock et al 1980, Upton 1985). The most common pattern (80%)

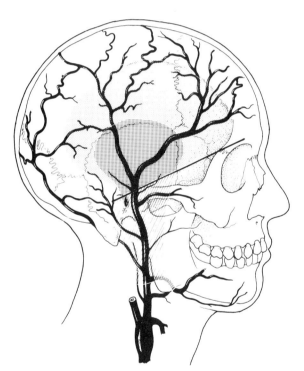

Fig. 9.3 The depth and location of the superficial temporal vessels varies. At the level of the external auditory meatus directly above the parotid gland (striped region) the vessels lie deep within the subcutaneous fat plane, where they are easily identified. Vessel identification is easiest at or above the meatus (heavily stippled) where the artery and vein(s) lie on top of the temporoparietal fascia. Superiorly (lightly stippled) dissection becomes quite difficult as the fascia is closer and more adherent to the overlying scalp. Initial vascular identification should be in the heavily stippled area. Note the bifurcation within 2.0 cm of the zygoma.

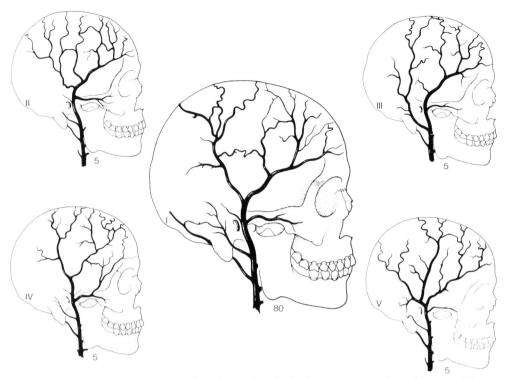

Fig. 9.4 The superficial temporal artery is the last major arborization of the external carotid system. Five major branching patterns are depicted, with the most common (80%) in the centre. These vessels are always found external to the temporoparietal fascia. The major arborization of the superficial temporal artery into anterior (frontal) and posterior (parietal) is within 2.0 cm of the zygoma. Note other branches which include the zygomaticomalar branch at the level of the zygoma, the anterior auricular branches at the level of the lobule of the ear, and the occipital artery which courses beyond the mastoid process of the temporal bone.

occurs with the major anterior (frontal) and posterior (parietal) bifurcation arising within 2.0 cm above the zygoma (Fig. 9.4). Proximal to this bifurcation, and usually below a line drawn between the external auditory meatus and the lateral orbital rim, lies the zygomaticomalar (zygomaticoorbital) branch of the superficial temporal artery, which runs transversely across the face. A reciprocal relationship often exists between this artery and the anterior bifurcation of the superficial temporal artery. When the zygomaticomalar vessel is large, a more distal bifurcation of the superficial temporal artery can be seen, and the anterior branch may be of smaller calibre. The opposite relationship may exist when the zygomaticomalar branch is small, with a very proximal take-off. In the preauricular region the middle temporal artery is often found on the underside of the superficial temporal artery, has an origin proximal to the zygomaticomalar branch,

and is often found within, or directly adjacent to, parotid tissue. This artery courses downwards along the fascia of the temporalis muscle (Abul-Hassan et al 1986), often called the deep temporal fascia. This is a fascial layer distinct from the temporoparietal fascia.

Other major branching patterns are seen with equal frequency (Fig. 9.4). The surgeon should be aware of their existence if wide extensions of fascia are planned in either direction, or if the fascia is to be divided into individual strips for use in different regions. The abundant anastomotic system carried by this fascia and delivering blood supply to the scalp is well known.

In most adults, and particularly elderly patients, redundant S-shaped tortuosities in the superficial temporal artery are common. This can be of clinical importance during the initial isolation of the STA and identification of major aborizations. In older individuals with these S-shaped configurations, the major axial artery may be initially identified lying in a transverse direction, and must be followed both proximal and distal to ensure its proper identification. No significant increase in intimal thickening, arteriosclerotic plaque formation or muscular hyperplasia has been seen in any of the author's adult patients or cadaver dissections. None of our patients have had collagen diseases such as temporal arteritis, but these conditions would make the use of this flap inadvisable.

Preauricular skin and scalp thickness is greater in hirsute males and thinner in children and elderly adults. Here, thick fibrous septa connect the fascia to the overlying scalp, which, as mentioned, becomes densely adherent above the crest of the temporal fossa. These connections become stretched and attenuated in older persons. No positive correlations are present between arterial branching patterns, internal vessel calibre and male pattern baldness. A very generous subcutaneous fat layer is found between the dermis of the preauricular skin and the temporoparietal fascia, often called the SMAS by the cosmetic surgeon, who may plicate this during facelift procedures (Jost & Ceuet 1984). The tremendous mobility of the temporal and frontal scalp and preauricular skin is made possible by the smooth areolar undersurface of the fascia, which glides over the adjacent fascia of the temporalis muscle.

DONOR FLAP ELEVATION

The preauricular and temporal scalp regions are judiciously shaved to allow for a 'T'or 'Y' extension well within the temporal scalp area (Fig. 9.5A). Appropriate modifications should be made for men whose biological fathers demonstrate a male pattern baldness distribution. The preauricular portion of the incision is made in the anterior crease, with a V-shaped extension above the tragus of the ear. The superficial temporal artery, with its major anterior (frontal) and posterior (parietal) bifurcations, is identified either by palpation or with a Doppler probe. Injections of saline with adrenaline are given in the hair-bearing scalp regions to decrease intradermal bleeding. The preauricular incision is made and the superficial

temporal artery and its accompanying vein are identified by blunt dissection. The auriculotemporal nerve is easily identified running longitudinally in front of the ear. Anterior and posterior scalp flaps with subcutaneous fat and hair follicles are then raised in an antegrade fashion. Thin flaps should be avoided, or hair follicles may be damaged. As elevation progresses towards the crest of the temporal fossa, the scalp flap dissection becomes much more tedious because of the closer relationship of the fascia and the overlying dermis of the scalp (see Fig. 9.1). Bipolar microvascular cauteries or hand-held battery-powered units are useful to control bleeding in this region, where abundant vascular channels are present. *If the scalp flaps are initially raised from above downwards, the temporoparietal fascia may inadvertently be included with the scalp flap.* It is recommended that the vessels should first be identified and the flap raised from below upwards.

At or above the level of the zygoma, near the lateral orbital rim, a nerve stimulator is helpful for identification of both orbital and frontal branches of the facial (VIIth) nerve, but these nerves *always* lie deep to the flap.

After the scalp flaps have been reflected, a precise template for flap size is obtained from the hand, where a second surgical team has simultaneously prepared the recipient site for the flap transfer. This may commonly include adjunctive procedures such as debridements, osteotomies, bone grafts and tendon grafts. The template is placed over the fascia with the axial vessel near its anterior margin. Most flaps do not exceed 8.0 cm in width and 14.0 cm in length. If additional width is required, extension into the posterior (parietal) portion of the field is recommended in deference to the anterior (frontal) margin, where fascial thickness is variable. The fascia is then incised along its superior and posterior borders and the flap is easily elevated in a retrograde fashion. The anterior border is incised under direct vision to avoid any nerve damage. This elevation is in the same plane which would be used for the 'Gillies' approach, for elevation of a depressed zygomatic fracture. The operator is often surprised by both the abundance and the calibre of the scalp vessels at or above the crest of the temporal fossa. For large flaps the auriculotemporal nerve should be

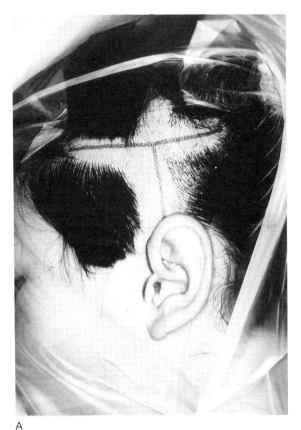

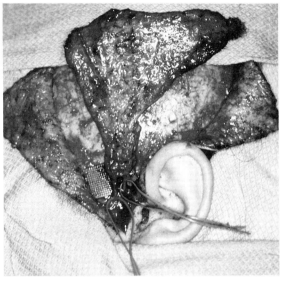

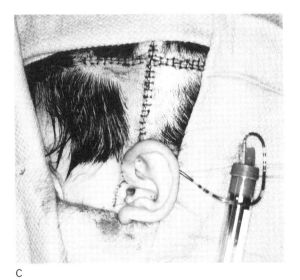

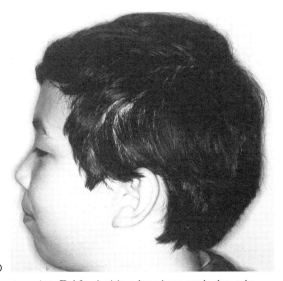

Fig. 9.5 Dissection: **A** Hair is shaved well within the hair-bearing scalp region. **B** After incisions have been made the scalp, flaps are dissected off the temporoparietal fascia. The fascial flap has been isolated as a vascular island. If extra tissue is needed, extension in a posterior (occipital) direction is recommended. **C** Scalp closure over a small suction drain. **D** Donor site 2 months later.

sacrificed. The fan-shaped flap then funnels down to its axial vessels, which have been isolated in front of the tragus of the ear (Fig. 9.5B).

If additional pedicle length is needed, more proximal isolation and dissection through the upper portion of the parotid gland can be carried out. In this region many vessels may be encountered, including anterior auricular arteries (0.4–1.0 mm), the zygomaticomalar (or transverse facial) vessels (0.4–1.8 mm), the anterior auricular branches of the superficial temporal artery, and the middle temporal artery (0.4–1.0 mm). Abnormal branching patterns of the STA should always be considered with dissections in this region (see Fig. 9.3). The middle temporal branch of the superficial temporal artery consistently arborizes in the region of the external auditory meatus on the deep surface of the STA, and may cause difficulty in passing circumferential ligatures around the STA. Abul Hassan et al (1986) have described the elevation of the temporalis muscle fascia as a separate fascial flap connected to the temporoparietal fascial flap. Following isolation as a vascular island, the flap is now ready for transfer.

Artery and vein are separated from one another to facilitate subsequent identification prior to vascular anastomoses.

COMPLICATIONS

Very few complications have been encountered with the author's use of this free tissue transfer in the hand. A two-team approach has been employed in all cases and operating time has generally been between 3 and 6 hours, depending upon the complexity of the recipient site reconstruction. Most complications relate to the critical flap elevation. If a rapid retrograde scalp dissection is performed high in the temporal scalp, the fascia may be included with the scalp flaps. Bleeding or careless dissection in and around the lateral canthus of the eye along the zygomatic arch may cause injury to the vulnerable frontalis branches of the facial nerve. Deep dissections within the parotid gland may result in haematoma or subsequent salivary fistulae. Thin anterior scalp flaps may cause alopecia. Although the scalp and preauricular incisions are very well concealed (Fig. 9.5C,D), they can be noticeable with certain types of haircut, (Fig. 9.6A). Although the auriculotemporal nerve is sometimes sacrificed with the flap, none of our patients have complained of altered sensation or dysaesthesia. Gustatory sweating (Frey's syndrome) has not been seen when proximal extensions of the dissection have been necessary to increase pedicle length.

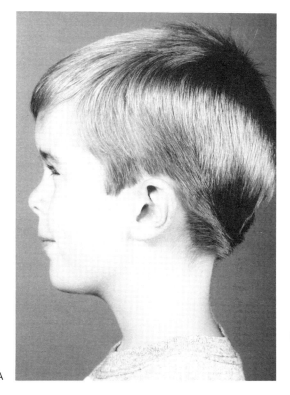

A

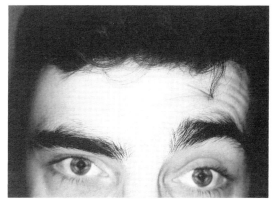

B

Fig. 9.6 A The scar is visible only with short haircuts. **B** Injury to the frontalis branch of facial (VIIth) nerve occurred in one patient.

The most serious problem which can occur from this donor flap elevation is injury to the frontal, orbital or zygomatic branches of the facial nerve (Fig. 9.6B). This did occur in one patient and has actually been the only problem the author has encountered with the temporoparietal fascial free flap. With proper traction and countertraction, a thin white line between the fascia of the scalp is represented by areolar tissue. Dissection within this plane easily separates the two. The same anatomic layer exists deep to the fascia, where elevation in a relatively bloodless field should be easily accomplished.

ADVANTAGES AND DISADVANTAGES

The advantages of the free parietotemporal fascial flap for acute and secondary hand reconstructions are numerous, and include large axial vessels (1.0–2.2 mm arterial diameter) with predictable anatomy, a satisfactory vascular pedicle (3.0–4.0 cm) and minimal donor-site morbidity. The donor-site dissection is straightforward but meticulous, and is completed in 1–1.5 hours. The donor-site scar is hidden. A two-team approach is possible, with one team working on the scalp and a second team preparing the extremity recipient site. No intraoperative positional changes are necessary. The fascial tissue is thin and pliable and can be isolated into segments which follow the vascular arborizations; this is convenient for use within web commissures and along adjacent sides of digits. The areolar underside of the fascia provides a potential gliding surface for tendons, and the overlying external surface provides an excellent bed for a split-thickness skin graft. The author has used fascia alone in the hand to reconstruct retinacula, or has covered it with split-thickness skin grafts for external resurfacing. The inclusion of segments of cortical or cortico-cancellous segments of temporal bone as a 'vascularized' bone graft is probably not justified in hand reconstruction. Anatomical dissections have not demonstrated that the major blood supply to the bone traverses this fascial layer; in fact, craniofacial reconstructions in which temporal bone has been used as a vascularized pedicle graft have included the temporalis muscle and its fascia, and there is no evidence at present that cranial bone grafts attached to temporoparietal fascia are vascularized.

The major disadvantage of this free tissue transfer is its relatively restricted size. The largest flap used by the author has been 10.5 cm × 14.5 cm, which has been large enough to resurface the dorsum of an adult hand in the metacarpal region, the dorsum of the foot, the entire heel or a small segment of an Achilles tendon. Some clinicians have reported partial fascial flap necrosis anteriorly, where the fascial thickness is predictably thin. If additional flap width is needed, extension should be made in a posterior or parietal direction (Fig. 9.5D). Potential complications have been listed, the most serious of which is injury to the frontal or orbital branches of the facial nerve. The additional time required for this or any free tissue transfer for acute and secondary hand reconstruction may be inappropriate for the patient with associated injuries or medical problems.

We prefer to transfer this distant source of vascularized fascia instead of local forearm fascia raised as a pedicle flap on the radial artery for several reasons. The latter forearm donor site gives a more conspicuous scar; donor-site dissection cannot be performed simultaneously by a second surgical team, and arterial input to the limb is reduced. Although the radial artery is not the dominant vessel to the hand in most individuals, incomplete communication between the radial and ulnar systems through the superficial and deep arches does exist, and in northern climates cold intolerance is more than a theoretic consideration (Coleman & Anson 1961). No large clinical series of forearm (Chinese) flaps has reported follow-up data on cold intolerance in distal circulation (Song & Song 1982). As a safety measure the author has always revascularized the radial artery when this tissue has been transferred as a free flap to some other part of the body.

CLINICAL CASE APPLICATIONS

The use of free vascularized fascial flaps provides no panacea, but is certainly both useful and practical in acute and secondary hand reconstruction. The author's initial applications were in situations

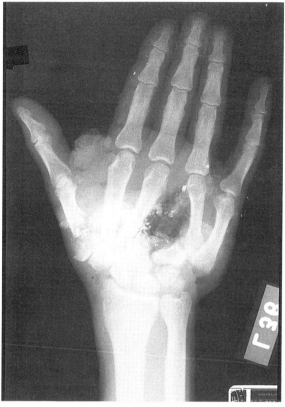

A

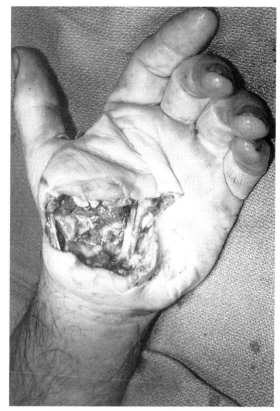

B

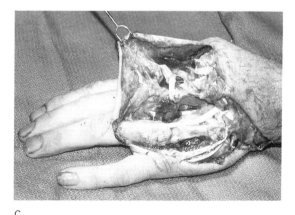

C

Fig. 9.7 A X-ray of a 47-year-old mine worker following a crush injury due to a mining accident. Comminuted fractures and/or dislocations are present at the carpometacarpal level of all digits and the thumb. **B, C** Extensive soft-tissue injury was present on both sides of the hand. **D** X-ray of the hand following open reduction, tendon repair and debridement. After 4 days the index ray was amputated and delayed primary closure of the wound was required. **E, F** A temporoparietal fascial flap (12.0 cm x 14.0 cm) was isolated as a vascular island, transferred and joined end-to-side to the radial artery on the palmar side of the wrist, passed through the index metacarpal defect and used to resurface the dorsum of the hand. **G, H** Appearance 14 months later. Sensation is intact. Total range of motion is poor, but the patient has a good thumb-long finger pinch. (Courtesy of William Swartz, MD.)

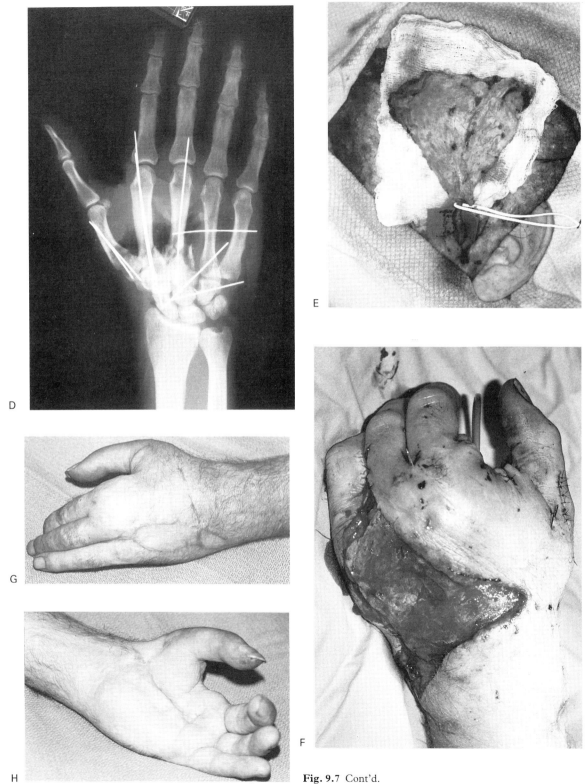

D

E

F

G

H

Fig. 9.7 Cont'd.

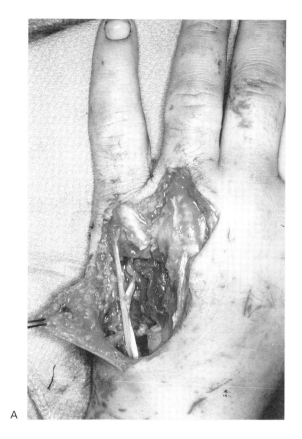

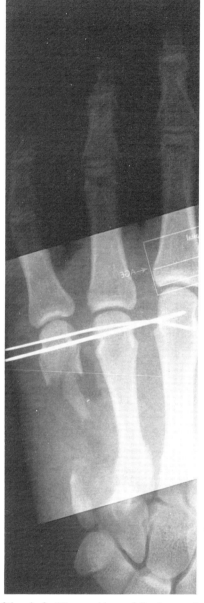

Fig. 9.8 Acute trauma with bone-graft reconstruction. **A** Appearance of the left hand of a 28-year-old man following crush injury in a roll-over motor vehicle accident. Injuries included subtotal loss of skin, tendon, interosseous muscle and fifth metacarpal. **B** X-ray shows subtotal metacarpal deficit. **C** Reconstruction consisted of an autogenous bone graft which was resurfaced with a vascularized temporoparietal flap joined end-to-side to the ulnar artery in Guyon's canal exposed through a palmar incision. The flap is seen prior to skin grafting. **D** Appearance of bone graft 14 months later. **E, F** Good extension of the fifth finger was maintained 18 months later. The patient returned to work 1 month post-injury. **G** Appearance of donor site. (Reproduced with permission of the Journal of Hand Surgery.)

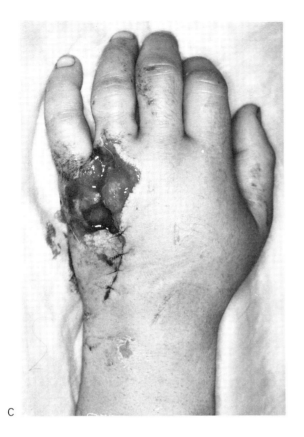

C

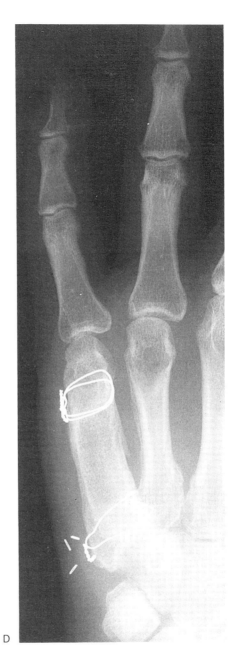

D

Fig. 9.8 Cont'd.

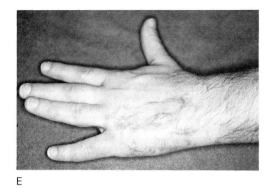

E

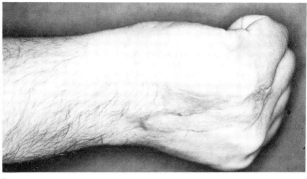

F

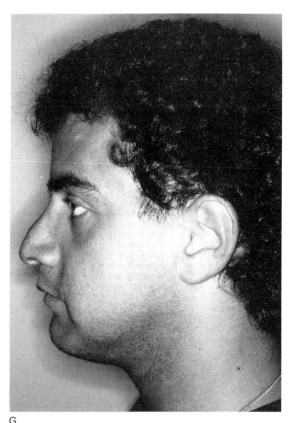

G

Fig. 9.8 Cont'd.

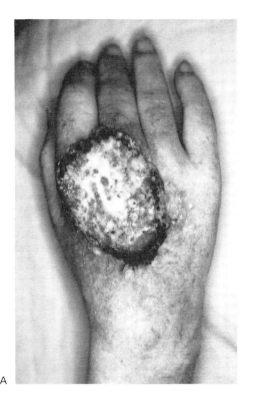

A

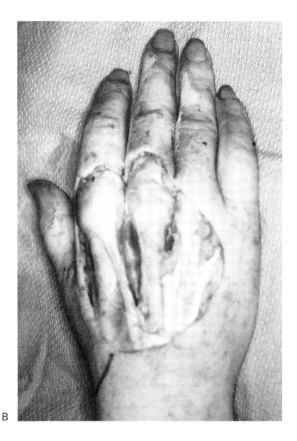

B

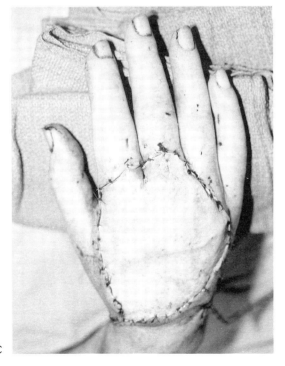

C

Fig. 9.9 Resurfacing the dorsum of the hand. **A** Chronic wound due to indolent squamous cell carcinoma in a 54-year-old electrician, which had been present for 6 years. **B** Resection included the tumour, adjacent skin, the common extensors to the index and long fingers as well as periosteum and interosseous muscles. **C** The defect was resurfaced with a 12.0 cm × 9.5 cm temporoparietal flap revascularized end-to-side to the radial artery and one vena comitans; the vascularized fascia was covered with a split-thickness skin graft. The flap was monitored with a Doppler directly over the skin graft. **D, E** Appearance 24 months later. The skin is mobile and supple. The patient has not elected to have the missing extensor reconstructed. He is back at work. (Reproduced in part with the permission of the Journal of Plastic and Reconstructive Surgery.)

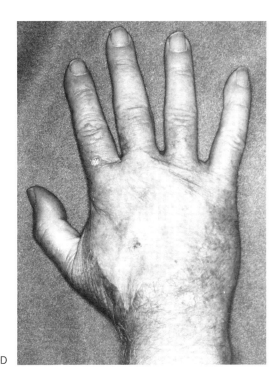

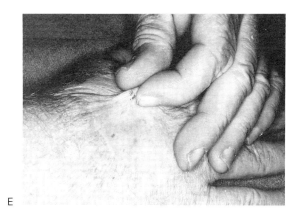

E

D

Fig. 9.9 Cont'd.

where small amounts of tissue were needed in critical regions to cover tendons, nerves, bones or joints. Despite our particular interest in the temporoparietal free flap, they constitute only 5% of our free flap transfers. The potential of the smooth areolar inner surface of the fascia for gliding of adjacent tendons is intriguing. The biological properties of the mesenchymal cells within the areolar gliding plane on the underside of the flap have not been studied in as much detail as have similar cells within the paratenon of tendons. Histologically they appear to be fibrocytes, with loose cellular connections and minimal adjacent vascularity. Tendon gliding has been preserved when this layer has been placed directly over the extensor and flexor tendons of the hand. Secondary extensor tendon grafts have been performed beneath fascial flaps used initially for dorsal hand resurfacing.

Our initial clinical uses of this free flap in the upper extremity were on the dorsum of the hand and fingers, and these eventually extended to more difficult regions on the palmar surface of the hand and within web spaces (Upton 1985). This thin tissue is most applicable in areas where small amounts of thin, pliable tissue are needed. When large amounts of tissue have been required, we have preferred to use other donor sites in single-stage free tissue transfers, but still frequently employ pedicle flaps from the groin or abdomen when free flap donor areas are not available or are contraindicated by medical problems.

Preoperative angiography has not been necessary if adequate donor vessels are easily identifiable on Doppler examination. For patients requiring secondary reconstructions in distal portions of the hand beyond the wrist, recipient site angiograms have frequently been obtained. Our initial applications following trauma have been extended for use in congenital vascular malformations, reconstruction of the insufficient thumb–index web space, resurfacing after tumour resection, burn reconstruction, and provision of a gliding bed following extensive tenolysis (Figs 9.7–9.12).

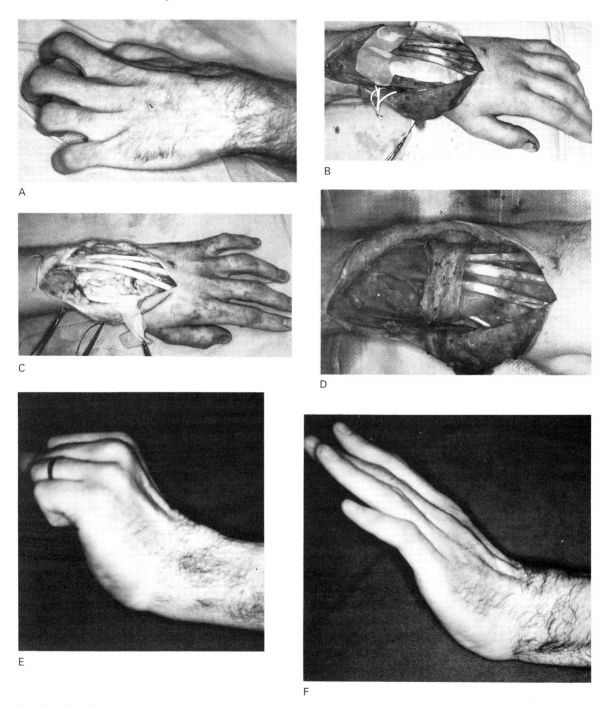

Fig. 9.10 Provision of vascular bed following tenolysis. **A** Patient attempting to make a fist 2 years after a severe crush injury: intrinsic tendons are tight and all soft tissue is adherent in a common scar, following three dorsal tenolyses and joint-release procedures. **B** Following excision of all scar tissue, no dorsal retinaculum or wrist capsule remains. The thumb extensor is not in continuity. **C** The rubber template shows the placement of two sections of temporoparietal fascia: one to reconstruct the dorsal wrist capsule and the other to create a vascularized dorsal retinaculum. **D** The fascia has been split between the arborizations of the anterior (frontal) and posterior (parietal) branches of the superficial temporal artery. Following revascularization the fascia is secured to bone. The smooth layer of the fascia is adjacent to the tendons. **E, F** Flexion and extension of wrist and digits 20 months postoperatively, with minimal bowstringing.

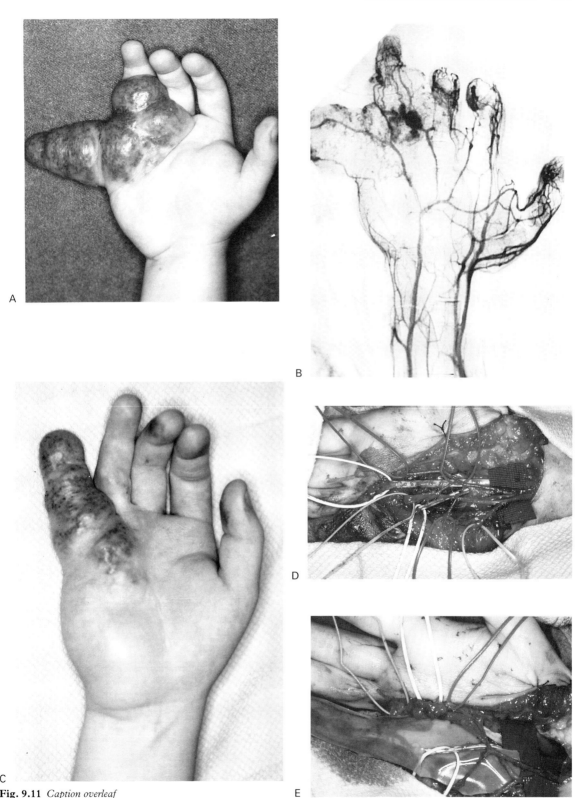

Fig. 9.11 *Caption overleaf*

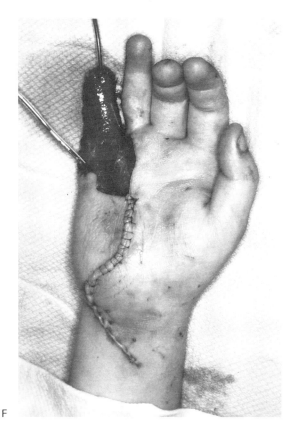

F

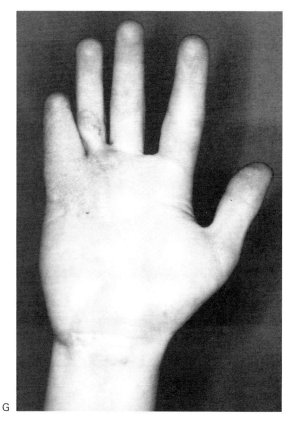

G

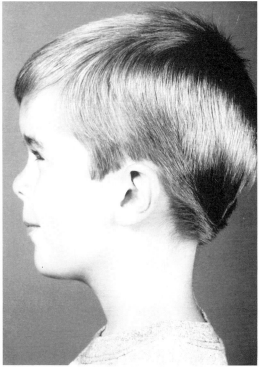

H

Fig. 9.11 Congenital malformation. **A** Appearance of a congenital low-flow vascular malformation in a 2-year-old child. **B** Angiogram showed no high-flow shunts as large venous lakes predominated. Arterial anatomy was normal. The extent of midpalmar malformation is not visualized well in this film. **C** Reconstruction consisted of staged excisions at yearly intervals. Appearance after the first staged debulking of the radial half of the palm and the ring finger. The fifth finger and hypothenar region have not been dissected and excess skin from the dorsum of the ring finger has been used to resurface its palmar side. **D** One year later the entire hypothenar region was dissected with excision of all involved skin. The flexor tendons are completely exposed in the midpalm. The background outlines the ulnar artery leading to the deep palmar arch and the ulnar nerve. All veins have been completely removed. **E** The template shows the position of the vascularized fascia which will be joined end-to-side to the ulnar artery and end-to-end to a subcutaneous vein pedicled from the radial side of the wrist. The terminal endings of the sensory nerves to the fifth finger are located deep to the fascia. The flexor tendon penetrates and runs deep to the fascia beyond the midpalm. **F** Appearance of vascularized fascia before application of a split-thickness skin graft. **G** Appearance 2 years later. Protective sensibility is present within the skin-grafted portion of the flap. Although two-point discrimination is greater than 12 mm, the patient has had no cuts, abrasions or bruises. **H** Donor-site appearance. (Reproduced in part with permission of the Journal of Hand Surgery.)

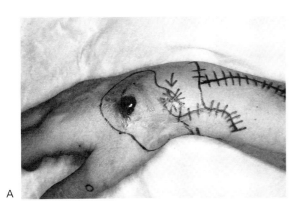

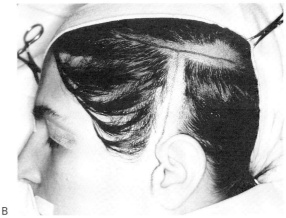

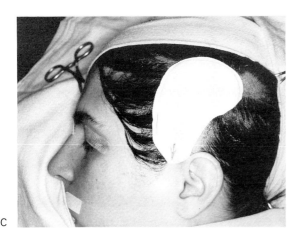

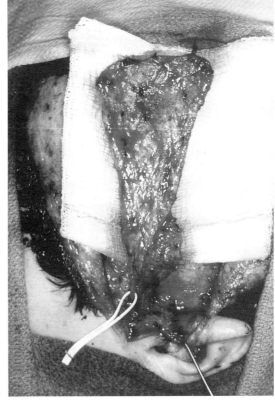

Fig. 9.12 Resurfacing chronic granuloma and neuromas. **A** Appearance of hand when patient presented with an unstable scar and a chronic granuloma 3 years after eight operations for neuromas in the dorsal sensory branches of the radial nerve. Initially the problem was related to a release of the first dorsal compartment. The outlines of multiple previous incisions are marked. There is no sensation in the dorsum of the hand. **B** Outline of 'T' incision in temporal scalp, and preauricular extension. **C** Template for tissue required. **D** Temporoparietal fascia isolated as a vascular island.
E Flap and template. **F** Appearance of the first and third compartments following extensive excision of scar. Multiple neuromas are seen over the background. **G** Following autogenous sural nerve grafts and extensor tenolysis. **H** The fascia has been revascularized with end-to-side anastomosis to the radial artery and one vena comitans. **I** Following skin-graft coverage.
J Appearance 12 months later. Protective sensibility has returned to the hand. There has been no loss of extensor tendon function following tenolysis. The patient has returned to work.

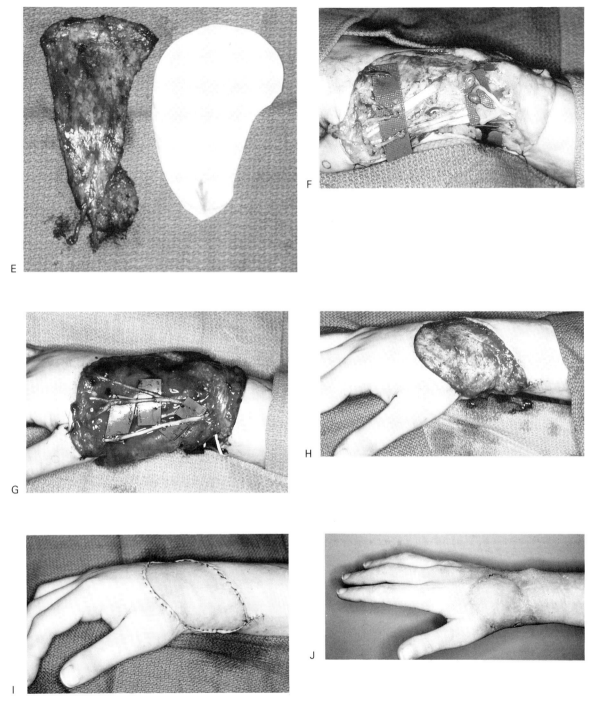

Fig. 9.12 Cont'd.

REFERENCES AND FURTHER READING

Abul-Hassan H S, Ascher G von D, Acland R D 1986 Surgical anatomy and blood supply of the fascial layers of the temporal region. Plastic and Reconstructive Surgery 77: 17

Adache B 1928 Das arterien system der Japaner. Verkagkaiser, Kyoto

Al-Kayat A, Bramley P 1979 A modified preauricular approach to the temporomandibular joint and malar arch. British Journal of Oral Surgery 17: 91

Avelar J J, Psillaris J M 1981 The use of galea flaps in craniofacial deformities. Annals of Plastic Surgery 6: 464

Brent B, Byrd H S 1983 Secondary ear reconstruction with cartilage grafts covered by axial, random and free flaps of temporoparietal fascia. Plastic and Reconstructive Surgery 72: 141

Brent B, Upton J, Acland R D et al 1985 Experience with the temporoparietal free flap. Plastic and Reconstructive Surgery 76: 177

Byrd H S 1980 The use of subcutaneous axial fascial flaps in reconstruction of the head. Annals of Plastic Surgery 4: 191

Cauldwell E W, Anson B J 1945 The surgical anatomy of the facial nerve. Surgery Gynecology and Obstetrics 80: 620

Coleman S S, Anson B J 1961 Arterial patterns in the hand based on a study of 650 specimens. Surgery Gynecology and Obstetrics 113: 409

Couly G, Hureau J, Valliane J M 1975 Le fascia superficialis cephalique. Annales de Chirurgie 20: 171

D'All Aiqua U 1901 Artère temporale superficielle chez l'homme. Acta Italica Biologica 36

Erol O O, Parsh F D, Spira M 1981 The use of the secondary island graft-flap reconstruction of the burned ear. British Journal of Plastic Surgery 34: 417

Eustathiasos N 1932 Etude anatomique sur les temporales superficielles. Annals of Anatomy and Pathology 9: 684

Fox J W, Edgerton M T 1976 The fan flap: an adjunct to ear reconstruction. Plastic and Reconstructive Surgery 58: 663

Harii K, Ohmori K, Ohmori A 1974 Hair transplantation with free scalp flap. Plastic and Reconstructive Surgery 53: 410

Jost G, Ceuet Y 1984 Parotid fascia and face lifting: a critical evaluation of the SMAS concept. Plastic and Reconstructive Surgery 74: 42

Lovie M J, Duncan, G M, Glasson D W 1984 The ulnar artery forearm free flap. British Journal of Plastic Surgery 37: 486

Mitz V, Peyronie M 1976 The superficial musculoaponeurotic system (SMAS) in the parotid and cheek area. Plastic and Reconstructive Surgery 58: 80

Monks G 1898 Restoration of a lower eyelid by a new method. Boston Medical and Surgical Journal 139: 385

Ohmori S 1978 Reconstruction of microtia using the silastic frame. Clinical Plastic Surgery 5: 379

Pitanguy I, Silveira R 1966 The frontal branch of the facial nerve: the importance of its variations in face lifting. Plastic and Reconstructive Surgery 38: 21

Quain R 1844 The anatomy of the arteries of the human body. Taylor and Walton, London

Ricbourg B, Mitz V, Lassau J P 1975 Artère temporale superficielle étude anatomique et déductions pratiques. Annales de Chirurgie 20: 197

Salmon 1936 Artères de la peau. Masson, Paris, p. 104

Smith R A 1980 The free fascial scalp flap. Plastic and Reconstructive Surgery 66: 204

Song R, Gao Y, Song Y 1982 The forearm flap. Clinical Plastic Surgery 9: 21

Song Y G, Chen G Z, Song Y L 1984 The free thigh flap: a new free flap based on the septocutaneous artery. British Journal of Plastic Surgery 37: 149

Stock A L, Collins H P, Davidson T M 1980 Anatomy of the superficial temporal artery. Head and Neck Surgery 2: 466

Tegtmeier R E, Goddins R A 1977 The use of a fascial flap in ear reconstruction. Plastic and Reconstructive Surgery 60: 406

Upton J 1985 Discussion: surgical anatomy of the temporal region. Plastic and Reconstructive Surgery 77: 25

Upton J 1988 Clinical applications of vascularized fascial flaps. In: Brunelli G, Textbook of Microsurgery. Masson, Milano, p 873–885

Upton J, Rogers C, Durham-Smith G, Swartz W M 1986 Clinical applications of free temporo-parietal flaps in hand reconstruction. Journal of Hand Surgery 11A: 475

Walton R L, Bunkis, J 1984 The posterior calf fasciocutaneous free flap. Plastic and Reconstructive Surgery 74: 76

David M. Evans and David Gault

10 Free flaps from the trunk and lower limb

The various situations in which free tissue transfer is used in hand resurfacing require a repertoire of donor sites (Chase 1984, Daniel & Faibisoff 1979, Daniel & Weiland 1982, Lister & Sheker 1988.) The most useful flaps are shown in Table 10.1. The osteocutaneous flaps and functioning gracilis flap are included for completeness, but will not be described in detail in this chapter because they are unlikely to be used primarily for resurfacing. The reader is referred to Webster & Soutar (1986), Gilbert (1981), Harrison (1986) and Manktelow & McKee (1978) for descriptions of these flaps.

FREE FLAPS FROM THE TRUNK

Latissimus dorsi flap

This is the most dependable and adaptable free-flap for large skin defects (Bailey 1979, Bailey & Godfrey 1982), and may be used as a myocutaneous flap (which tends to be bulky when used in the forearm and hand), as a muscle flap resurfaced with split skin, or as a functioning reinnervated muscle combined with resurfacing by either means. Shoulder function is not significantly impaired following its removal as a free flap (Laitung & Peck 1985). Latissimus dorsi has one dominant vascular pedicle which enters the muscle with the nerve about 10 cm from the humeral insertion. Often smaller vessels enter the muscle around its origin from the chest wall and through the undersurface, but the whole muscle and its overlying skin can survive on the main pedicle (Bartlett et al 1981). A 10 cm pedicle can be prepared by dividing side branches up to the origin of the thoracodorsal artery and the vein from the axillary artery and vein. The two main branches are the subscapular artery and the artery to serratus anterior, with accompanying veins (Fig. 10.1).

Before the flap is raised, the free lateral edge of the muscle should be marked on the skin with the patient awake. Although the muscle can be dissected with the patient supine, propped up with sandbags, it is much easier in the lateral position, and if skin is to be included this is essential. The arm is placed on a high, padded support to expose the axilla widely, taking care not to exert traction on the brachial plexus (Logan & Black 1985). Dissection starts on the lateral free edge of the muscle, and the submuscular plane is identified below the point of entry of the pedicle. This plane is developed easily beneath the whole free portion of the muscle. Retraction of the muscle now re-

Table 10.1 Free-flap donor sites for the upper limb

Tissue	Size	Donor site
Skin	Small	Lateral arm flap
		Medial arm flap
		Scapular flap
		Temporoparietal fascia + skin
Skin + innervation	Small	Custom-made big-toe flap
		Dorsalis pedis flap
Skin + tendon	Small	Dorsalis pedis flap (can be innervated)
Skin	Large	Groin flap (SCIA)
		Latissimus dorsi myocutaneous flap
		Latissimus dorsi muscle + SSG
		Contralateral radial forearm flap
Skin + functioning muscle	Large	Innervated latissimus dorsi + skin or SSG
		Gracilis
Skin & bone	Large or small	DCIA + iliac crest
		Fibular osteocutaneous flap

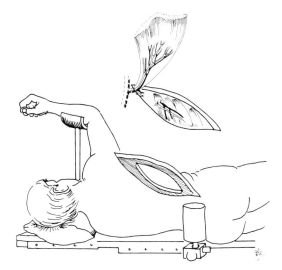

Fig. 10.1 The patient positioned for dissection of a latissimus dorsi flap. Care is needed not to apply upward traction on the arm, to avoid damage to the brachial plexus, and the arm should be kept in front of the coronal plane for the same reason. The muscle, with or without a paddle of skin, is dissected with the thoracodorsal vessels, and the branch to serratus anterior has to be divided as shown in the inset.

veals the pedicle, which is tethered to the chest wall by the branch to serratus anterior. This vessel is ligated, and the pedicle is dissected to the top of the axilla. The nerve to latissimus dorsi runs with the vessels. The vein may be single and large, or double, and needs careful dissection where it is to be divided, usually close to the axillary vein, together with the artery in order to provide substantial vessels for easy anastomosis. It is important to prepare adequate lengths of the vessels for ease of handling, and to mark them with different clamps when the time comes to divide them, immediately before transfer of the flap.

Once the pedicle has been prepared, the rest of the flap is raised. If an island of skin is to be included this is incised, and temporary sutures are placed to tether the skin to the muscle in order to avoid shearing. It is not safe to take a very small island of skin, as this reduces the likelihood of a vertical perforator from the muscle entering the flap, and particularly threatens venous drainage. The skin paddle should be 2 inches or more in diameter to be safe. More than one such paddle can be taken if necessary, or it may be irregularly shaped. Finally, the remaining skin is separated from the muscle, the lower and medial origins

of the muscle are divided, and the upper insertion is divided only when the flap is ready for transfer. This protects the pedicle from accidental traction.

If the muscle alone is being transferred, it is sutured under natural tension into the defect, preferably imbricating it under surrounding healthy skin. An unexpanded mesh graft is then sutured over it without a tie-over dressing. If skin is included, the muscle should be sutured in place before the skin is closed. In the case of a functioning transfer the nerve will have to be prepared with the pedicle to give adequate length, and should be sutured to a predominantly motor nerve, such as the anterior or posterior interosseous nerve in the forearm. Ensuring proximity to such a nerve for suture without tension is an essential part of planning. The muscle has to be sutured to its new origin, and to the tendon or tendons, under sufficient tension for it to act effectively, and this is the most difficult aspect of the repair. Some kind of tendon weave into the muscle is necessary. It is not difficult to revascularize the muscle and achieve active contraction, but to harness that contraction effectively with adequate tension and without adhesions is extremely difficult. A later tenolysis is likely to be necessary. An example of such a transfer is shown in Fig. 10.2A–E. If the skin overlying latissimus dorsi is included, it may be that a freer excursion of the muscle is obtained, but the flap is then very bulky.

Scapular flap

This flap is useful for fairly small defects, the maximum dimensions that will allow direct closure of the donor-site being 12 cm by up to about 25 cm. The skin is thick and the subcutaneous tissue firm but not too deep, and the pedicle can be extended up to the thoracodorsal artery, giving 10 mm length and good vessels (Barwick et al 1982, Gahos et al 1985, Gilbert & Teot 1982, Hamilton & Morrison 1982, Mayou et al 1982, Urbaniak et al 1982, Fissette & Lahaye 1983, Dos Santos 1984). The flap is usually raised as a horizontal ellipse crossing the scapula half way between the spine and the lower pole of the scapula (Fig. 10.3). The subscapular artery and vein emerge through the triangular space between

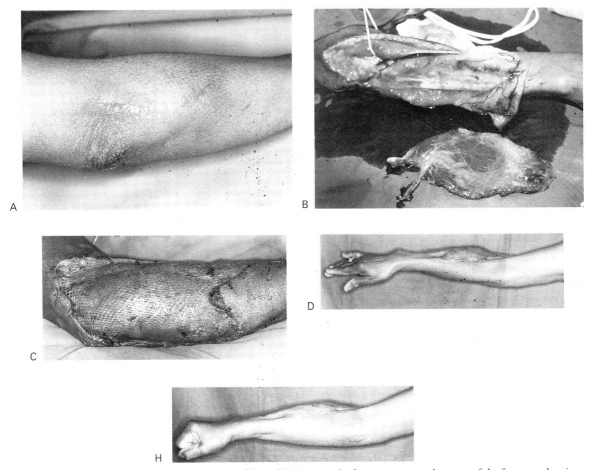

Fig. 10.2 A This patient has a recurrent malignant fibrous histiocytoma in the extensor muscle group of the forearm, showing the previous excision scar. **B** A compartment excision has been completed, preserving only extensor carpi radialis longus. Latissimus dorsi has been prepared, and clamps are seen on the artery and vein. **C** The muscle has been revascularized by end-to-side anastomosis to the brachial vessels, and the nerve sutured to the posterior interosseous nerve. The muscle has been attached to the lateral epicondyle, and distally to the extensor tendons under tension, and mesh-grafted. **D,E** One year later the muscle is seen functioning well – contraction (**D**) and relaxation (**E**) – and incidentally providing soft-tissue replacement.

triceps, teres major and the lateral margin of the scapula. As they emerge they turn laterally and run in a deep subcutaneous plane, giving branches to the skin. Elevation of the flap commences medially; it is important to develop the plane of dissection deep to all layers of the superficial fascia, since it is possible to raise the flap *too* superficial to include the supplying vessels. As the flap is raised towards its lateral end, vessels will be seen running in its deep surface, and can be traced to their emergence at the triangular space. If an extended pedicle is required, the large branch to the subscapularis muscle has to be ligated and the vessels traced through into the axilla, which has

to be dissected as for the pedicle of a latissimus dorsi flap.

The donor defect is closed directly, with undermining as necessary. The parascapular flap may be aligned obliquely downwards from the same vascular pedicle (Nassif et al 1982, Fissette & Lahaye 1983). An extended flap can be raised, but this leaves a defect that requires grafting, which may not be satisfactory over the mobile scapula.

Groin flap

Although it was one of the first free-flap donor

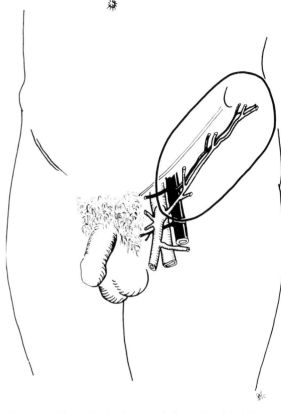

Fig. 10.4 The groin flap is centred along a line 1 in below and parallel to the inguinal ligament. The vessels are small and subject to some variation in their precise position of origin.

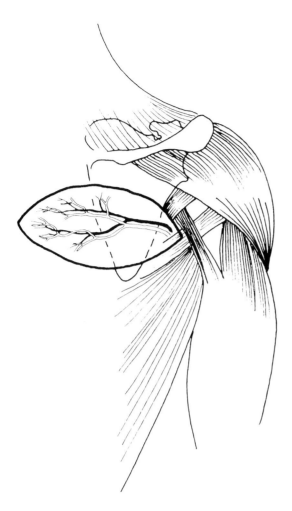

Fig. 10.3 The scapular flap is centred over the circumflex scapular vessels, half way down the lateral border of the scapula. The pedicle can be elongated by dissecting through into the axilla.

sites to be described (Daniel & Taylor 1973, Baudet et al 1976), the groin has to some extent been superseded by other donor sites. The one big advantage is the possibility of direct closure even after removal of a flap 15 cm or more in width, and the relatively concealed donor site. The amount of fat present varies according to body build, but the pedicle end has to carry some fat, and the main disadvantages of the flap are the shortness of the pedicle compared to other flaps, and the small calibre of the superficial circumflex iliac vessels on which it is based. Taylor et al (1979a,b) suggested the use of the deep circumflex iliac vessels, which are larger and run a longer course, but their connection with the skin is more

tenuous and more lateral, and the flap is usually only used in conjunction with vascularized bone from the iliac crest – the 'DCIA' flap (Ohmori & Harii 1975). Even then, the circulation to the overlying skin is slower than one expects in other free flaps.

The groin flap based on the superficial circumflex iliac vessels (SCIA flap) still has a limited place when a fairly large area of skin is required in a patient who particularly wants a concealed donor scar. Because of the difficulty with the pedicle already mentioned, its placing and length need careful planning, and vein grafts may be required.

Because the superficial circumflex iliac vessels are subject to anomalies (Baudet et al 1976), it is wise to dissect their origin from the femoral artery and femoral or long saphenous vein before raising the flap. Once their presence and position have been established, the flap is raised from lateral to medial. The central longitudinal axis of the flap runs parallel to, and 1 in below, the inguinal ligament (Fig. 10.4), and the flap can extend medially to the line of the femoral artery, and laterally at least to the midlateral line, and, less reliably, beyond. Some marginal loss can be encountered beyond that line.

The lateral extremity of the flap may be raised without the full thickness of the subcutaneous fat, but as the dissection reaches the line of sartorius muscle, it is deepened through the deep fascia to expose the muscle. This ensures inclusion of the supplying vessels with the flap. At the medial angle of the fascial compartment containing sartorius, the fascia is again incised, taking the dissection into the adipose tissue overlying the femoral nerve. The vessels cross in this fat layer and can be dissected out of it to join the previous dissection of the vessel origins. Because they are so small they have to be very carefully prepared, making use of all available length, and carefully marked prior to division. When the flap has been raised it may be possible to tease some of the unwanted fat away from the vascular pedicle, but great care is needed to avoid damage to the vascular connections of the flap.

After removal of the flap the donor site can be closed by direct approximation of the skin without undermining, unless an enormous flap has been removed, in which case skin grafts could be needed. Usually the wound closes easily in the line of the groin crease, by flexing the hip to 90°. This position has to be maintained for several days postoperatively, the simplest method of achieving this being to bandage the knee in flexion, taking care to avoid pressure in the popliteal fossa or calf. After several days the patient is allowed to slowly extend the hip, a process that may take 10 days, after which full extension is restored.

FREE FLAPS FROM THE LOWER LIMB

Dorsalis pedis flap

This flap provides excellent skin for resurfacing the hand, with dependable vascular connections, but at the expense of a potentially troublesome adherent skin graft on the dorsum of the foot. Reinnervation can be produced by repair of the

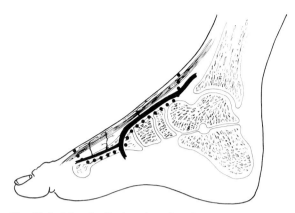

Fig. 10.5 A longitudinal section of the foot, showing the deep position of the dorsalis pedis artery and its distal branch, the first dorsal metatarsal artery; (these are indicated by the thick black line). The level of dissection is indicated by the dotted line, and has to be at the skeletal plane to keep the vessel with the skin.

superficial peroneal nerve to a local sensory nerve at the recipient site. The tendons of extensor digitorum longus can be included with the flap, surrounded by their intact vascularized gliding mechanisms, providing tendon grafts with a reduced tendency to adhesion formation. It is also possible to take the second metatarsal with the flap, but this increases the local donor-site problem. The flap is based on the dorsalis pedis artery and either the long saphenous vein, or a smaller superficial vein, or occasionally a vena comitans, although this is less reliable. The connection between the dorsalis pedis artery and the skin is through small perforating branches which pass superficially distal to the extensor retinaculum, and a conscious effort is needed during dissection to avoid transgression of the easily entered plane superficial to the artery. It is better to design the flap with some distal overlap beyond the point of deep departure of the dorsalis pedis artery, and to deliberately include some of the first dorsal metatarsal artery if this is placed superficially, since this artery may also provide some of the distal connections (Fig. 10.5). After outlining the margins of the flap the dissection starts with the isolation of the venous drainage and dissection of the required length of vein away from the flap. If needed, the superficial peroneal nerve and extensor digitorum longus tendons can also be isolated at the proximal and distal ends of the flap.

Deep dissection starts medially, beneath the

superficial veins, until the fascia carrying extensor hallucis longus tendon is encountered. This fascia is incised longitudinally, leaving enough fascia to cover the tendon prior to grafting, and the dissection is deepened vertically, lateral to the tendon, down to the periosteum over the cuboid. If this is not done carefully the plane between the dorsalis pedis artery and the skin is easily entered, and the flap will then be accidentally raised without its artery. Extensor hallucis brevis is encountered and divided as it runs obliquely across to join extensor hallucis longus tendon. By creeping laterally on the cuboid, the plane beneath the artery is opened and the artery can then be seen running with the flap. It is traced distally until it dives deeply between the bases of the first and second metatarsals, where it is ligated, keeping the first dorsal metatarsal artery as it runs distally, if the flap is to be extended distally. (Fig. 10.5).

The lateral side of the flap is now raised on the plane superficial to the fascia covering the long extensor tendons. As soon as the tendon to the second toe has been reached dissection again dives deeply, dividing the muscle belly of extensor digitorum brevis and lateral arterial branches on the way, entering the plane deep to the dorsalis pedis artery as in the medial dissection. The flap should now be ready to be lifted out of its bed when the last distal connections have been divided. The dissection of the dorsalis pedis artery is continued upwards until the desired length has been reached. If this is extended much above the ankle the collateral circulation round the ankle is compromised, and extension of the artery with a vein graft is preferable. If the extensor tendons are to be included in the flap they are dissected carefully with their gliding mechanisms intact, and are divided proximally and distally to provide the requisite length.

After transfer of the flap the donor site is repaired by use of a thick split-skin graft. Before applying the graft, complete haemostasis is most important and the graft should be sutured very carefully in place and packed into all the deep crevices between the tendons, which must be covered with fascia. Inevitably a part of the graft will be directly on to the periosteum of the cuboid bone, and will be adherent at this point. Provided good graft-take is achieved this should not be troublesome, but any scarring or instability of the graft at this site can lead to crust formation and possibly breakdown of the skin graft over the long term.

Free flaps from the toes

The indications for innervated pulp flaps from the toes are mentioned in Chapter 15 on fingertip injuries by Foucher (p 186). A defect of finger or thumb can be reconstructed using composite tissues from the toe designed to replace whatever tissues are required, including bone, tendon and gliding mechanisms, joints, nail and innervated skin. The donor toe is usually the big toe, which can be preserved in a functional and cosmetically acceptable state, and the vascular pedicle is traced back to the dorsalis pedis artery and long saphenous vein, giving ample length (Buncke & Rose 1979, Doi & Hattori 1980, Foucher et al 1980, Morrison et al 1980).

REFERENCES AND FURTHER READING

Bailey B N 1979 Latissimus dorsi flap – a practical approach. Annals of the Academy of Medicine of Singapore 8: 445

Bailey B N, Godfrey A M 1982 Latissimus dorsi muscle free flaps. British Journal of Plastic Surgery 47: 35

Bartlett S P, May J W, Yaremchuk M J 1981 The latissimus dorsi muscle: a fresh cadaver study of the neurovascular pedicle. Plastic and Reconstructive Surgery 67: 631

Barwick W J, Goodkind D J, Serafin D 1982 The free scapular flap. Plastic and Reconstructive Surgery 69: 779

Baudet J, LeMaire J M, Guimberteau J C 1976 Ten free groin flaps. Plastic and Reconstructive Surgery 57: 577

Buncke H J, Rose E H 1979 Free toe-to-fingertip neurovascular flaps. Plastic and Reconstructive Surgery 63: 607

Chase R A 1984 The development of tissue transfer in hand surgery. Journal of Hand Surgery 9A: 467

Coleman J J, Jurkiewicz M J 1984 Methods of providing sensation to anaesthetic areas. Annals of Plastic Surgery 12: 177

Daniel R K, Faibisoff B 1979 Free flap transfers for upper extremity reconstruction. Annals of the Academy of Medicine of Singapore 8: 440

Daniel R K, Taylor G I 1973 Distant transfer of an island flap by microvascular arterial anastomosis: a clinical technique. Plastic and Reconstructive Surgery 52: 111

Daniel R K, Weiland A J 1982 Free tissue transfers for upper extremity reconstruction. Journal of Hand Surgery 7: 66

Daniel R K, Terzis J, Midgley R D 1976 Restoration of sensation to an anaesthetic hand by a free neurovascular flap from the foot. Plastic and Reconstructive Surgery 57: 275

Doi K, Hattori S 1980 Free neurovascular flap from the first web space of the foot for reconstruction of the mutilated hand. Hand 12: 130

Dos Santos L F 1984 The vascular anatomy and dissection of the free scapular flap. Plastic and Reconstructive Surgery 73: 599

Fissette J, Lahaye T et al 1983 The use of the free parascapular flap in mid-palmar soft-tissue defect. Annals of Plastic Surgery 10: 235

Foucher G, Merle M, Maneaud M, Michon J 1980 Microsurgical free partial toe transfer in hand reconstruction. Plastic and Reconstructive Surgery 65: 616

Gahos F N, Tross R B et al 1985 Scapular free-flap dissection made easier. Plastic and Reconstructive Surgery 75: 115

Gilbert A 1981 Free vascularized bone graft. International Surgery 66: 27

Gilbert A, Teot L 1982 The free scapular flap. Plastic and Reconstructive Surgery 69: 601

Hamilton S G A, Morrison W A 1982 The scapular free flap. British Journal of Plastic Surgery 35: 2

Harrison D H 1986 The osteocutaneous free fibular graft. Journal of Bone and Joint Surgery 68B : 804

Laitung J K G, Peck F 1985 Shoulder function following the loss of the latissimus dorsi muscle. British Journal of Plastic Surgery 38: 375

Lister G, Scheker L 1988 Emergency free flaps to the upper extremity. Journal of Hand Surgery 13A: 22

Logan A M, Black M J M 1985 Injury to the brachial plexus resulting from shoulder positioning during latissimus dorsi flap pedicle dissection. British Journal of Plastic Surgery 38: 380

McGraw J B, Furlow L T 1975 The dorsalis pedis arterialized flap. Plastic and Reconstructive Surgery 55: 177

Man D, Acland R D 1980 The microarterial anatomy of the dorsalis pedis free flap and its clinical applications. Plastic and Reconstructive Surgery 65: 419

Manktelow R T, McKee N H 1978 Free muscle transplantation to provide active finger flexion. Journal of Hand Surgery 3: 416

Mayou B J, Whitby D, Jones B M 1982 The scapular flap – an anatomical and clinical study. British Journal of Plastic Surgery 35: 8

Morrison W A, O'Brien B M, MacLeod A M 1980 Thumb reconstruction with a free neurovascular wraparound from the big toe. Journal of Hand Surgery 5: 575

Morrison W A, O'Brien B McC, MacLeod A M, Gilbert A 1978 Neurovascular free flaps from the foot for innervation of the hand. Journal of Hand Surgery 3: 235

Nassif T M, Vidal L, Bovet J L, Baudet T 1982 The parascapular flap: a new cutaneous microsurgical free flap. Plastic and Reconstructive Surgery 69: 591

O'Brien B M 1985 Microvascular surgery of the upper extremity. Journal of Hand Surgery 10A: 982

Ohmori K, Harii K 1975 Free groin flaps: their vascular basis. British Journal of Plastic Surgery 28: 238

Ohmori K, Harii K 1976 Free dorsalis pedis sensory flap to the hand, with microneurovascular anastomoses. Plastic and Reconstructive Surgery 58: 546

Robinson D W 1976 Microsurgical transfer of the dorsalis pedis neurovascular island flap. British Journal of Plastic Surgery 29: 209

Shah K G, Garrett J C, Buncke H J 1979 Free groin flap transfers to the upper extremity. Hand 11: 315

Strauch B, Tsur H 1978 Restoration of sensation to the hand by a free neurovascular flap from the first web space of the foot. Plastic and Reconstructive Surgery 62: 361

Takami H, Takashahi S et al 1983 Use of the dorsalis pedis free flap for reconstruction of the hand. Hand 15: 173

Taylor G I, Townsend P 1979 Composite free flap and tendon transfer. An anatomical study and a clinical technique. British Journal of Plastic Surgery 32: 170

Taylor G I, Townsend P, Corlett R 1979a Superiority of the deep circumflex iliac vessels as the supply for the free groin flap: experimental work. Plastic and Reconstructive Surgery 64: 595

Taylor G I, Townsend P, Corlett R 1979b Superiority of the deep circumflex iliac vessels as the supply for the free groin flap: clinical work. Plastic and Reconstructive Surgery 64: 745

Urbaniak J R, Koman L A, Goldner R G et al 1982 The vascularized cutaneous scapular flap. Plastic and Reconstructive Surgery 69: 772

Van Genechten A, Townsend P L G 1983 Free composite tissue transfer in a compound hand injury. Hand 15: 325

Webster M H C, Soutar D S 1986 Practical guide to free tissue transfer. Butterworths, London

Zuker R M, Manktelow R T 1986 The dorsalis pedis free flap. Plastic and Reconstructive Surgery 77: 93

Tsu-Min Tsai, Joanne Werntz, Marc Bissonnette and Warren Breidenbach

11 Venous free flaps

INTRODUCTION

During the past 15 years there has been rapid progress in free tissue transfer. With increased experience, what used to be a highly demanding and hazardous procedure has become standard and very reliable. Stimulated by the increasing clinical application of free tissue transfer, several teams have investigated the possibilities of flap survival based only on the restoration of venous circulation.

Since 1983, the authors have been involved in clinical and experimental studies of the venous flap; these studies and experience will be presented and discussed.

HISTORY

At the beginning of the century, Alexis Carrel (Carrel & Guthrie 1906) had the idea that tissue viability could be improved by retrograde arterial blood flow through the venous system. He applied this concept clinically. An arteriovenous fistula was created proximal to the ischaemic tissue in an ischaemic lower extremity, in the hope of improving tissue viability. In spite of some successful attempts, however, this procedure was eventually abandoned because of its unpredictability.

The concept of tissue survival based on venous circulation is now applied to free tissue transfer. At present, even though the physiology of the nutrient circulation in venous flaps is not fully understood, there is clinical evidence that the venous circulation can support tissue survival to a certain extent.

DEFINITION

A venous flap is a composite flap consisting of skin and subcutaneous veins, which are used to reestablish a nutrient circulation through the flap (Baek et al 1985, Ji et al 1984, Tsai et al 1987). The flap may contain a single vein or a rich venous plexus. An arterial network can also be present, but will not be used for revascularization of the flap.

To achieve revascularization of a venous flap there are several options. The inflow can be arterial, venous or both, with similar variations in the outflow (Nakayama et al 1981, Mundy & Panje 1984). The importance of these different types of circulation regarding the nutrition and survival of a venous flap is not yet completely understood. When the inflow to the flap has an arterial component we refer to an 'arterialized' venous flap, as opposed to a 'venous flap' where the inflow and outflow are venous.

EXPERIMENTAL VENOUS FLAPS

Experimental attempts have been made to elucidate the physiological basis of the venous flap. Baek et al (1985) reported that a large venous flap based on the saphenous venous system alone survived successfully in the dog, while the same tissue without any vascular connections (i.e. a composite graft) did not. In the authors' laboratory similar experiments were carried out using mongrel dogs. Twenty-nine venous saphenous flaps were created in 29 dogs, in the lower extremity. This flap was created by elevating the saphenous flap with only the venous inflow and outflow intact. The saphenous artery and nerve were transected proximal and distal to the flap. In contrast to the 100% survival observed by Baek et al with this flap, only four (13.5%) of the venous flaps survived for 2 weeks.

One explanation for the failure of the canine venous saphenous flap would be the limited venous plexus. In contrast to this, the cephalic vein in the foreleg of the dog forms a much larger venous plexus; a canine cephalic venous flap was therefore developed. This flap was positioned on the radial aspect of the volar forearm along the course of the cephalic vein. The flap was elevated containing all skin and subcutaneous tissue and fascia over the underlying muscle. The veins entering distally (cephalic and accessory cephalic) and one leaving proximally (cephalic) were preserved. All other structures were transected, thus creating a flap connected only by its proximal and distal veins.

Eight canine venous cephalic flaps were created and six survived (75%) for 2 weeks. It is possible that these cephalic venous flaps survived as a composite graft. In order to explore this possibility, eight cephalic composite grafts were created and returned to the original bed. Only one of these flaps survived (12.5%). The difference in survival rates between the cephalic venous flap and cephalic composite graft was statistically significant ($P = 0.04$ using the chi-squared test).

From these results it can be concluded that there are certain flaps which can survive on only venous inflow and outflow. It appears that the greater the venous plexus, the more likely the flap is to survive. The venous flap appears less hardy than a regular arterialized flap, but on the other hand, clearly survives more readily than a comparable composite graft.

Baek et al (1985) concluded that venous flaps survive on venous blood flow through the capillaries. In other words, the blood flow ran from vein to venule into capillaries, and then returned to the vein. Evidence for this retrograde flow is substantiated by venograms which appeared to show capillary flow. There were two assumptions in this conclusion, first that the venous valve system is absent or incompetent at the venule level, and second that oxygen extraction from capillaries

supplied with venous blood is sufficient to support the flaps.

There is some clinical evidence that the venous flaps do have capillary flow. Our clinical observation of venous flaps clearly demonstrates a pink colour, with the blanching and refill characteristic of capillary filling. The possibility of capillary venous flow in these flaps is currently being investigated in our laboratory through the use of radioactive microspheres.

INDICATIONS

The indications for the clinical use of venous flaps include small soft-tissue defects that are not amenable to skin grafting or closure by a local flap because of size, location or quality of the underlying tissue bed. There are two clinical situations in which venous flaps should be strongly considered:

1. In the event of a finger amputation or devascularization where there is loss of skin and a segmental defect in the vascular structure, a venous flap could be used to reestablish the venous drainage of the finger and to achieve soft-tissue closure without tension (Honda et al 1984).
2. A failing replant caused by venous congestion could also benefit from a venous flap. This will allow debridement of any marginal or contused skin, reconstruction of the venous system and closure without tension.

In both of the indications outlined above, vein grafts to reestablish either venous flow dorsally or arterial flow volarly, are harvested as a composite skin graft to maximize technical efficiency by reinstating vessel continuity simultaneously with coverage of the soft-tissue defect.

More recently, small defects of the hand have been covered by venous flaps with some success. As clinical experience increases, the indications may become more extensive.

TECHNIQUE

The defect to be covered is first débrided back to normal tissue. Veins at the site of the defect are exposed for 0.5 cm both proximally and distally, and a pattern of the defect is obtained. Depending on the amount of skin needed, the donor site is selected – usually the dorsum of an uninjured finger can provide a flap of 1 cm × 4 cm. For larger flaps the volar surface of the forearm or the dorsum of the foot will be chosen.

First the outline of the flap is marked. If the dorsum of a finger is chosen, the flap boundaries should not exceed the midlateral line laterally and the metacarpophalangeal and distal interphalangeal joint at each end. The subcutaneous veins are exposed at each end over a segment large enough to allow length for venous reconstruction.

The flap, including skin, subcutaneous tissue and veins, is raised en bloc in the areolar plane just above the paratenon. The donor defect is later reconstructed using a full- or split-thickness skin graft held in place by a tie-over dressing. The flap is then transferred to the defect and the venous anastomoses are done. Usually two to three anastomoses are performed both proximally and distally to establish a flow-through pattern. The edge of the flap is then sutured loosely.

A soft-tissue dressing and splint are applied, leaving part or all of the flap exposed for clinical evaluation. The flap is monitored hourly by capillary refill, colour change and temperature.

Anticoagulant therapy is not used routinely, but in the early postoperative period most patients are given 80 mg of aspirin daily. Smoking is not permitted during the first 3 weeks following surgery. In the immediate postoperative period special attention must be directed towards the early detection of haematoma formation under the flap. This complication, if not treated promptly, can lead to loss of the flap due to either vessel spasm or excessive compression at the anastomosed site leading to failure of the anastomosis or secondary infection of the haematoma. For this reason, it is very important that the flap is sutured in place loosely, allowing fluid drainage between the stitches.

When the flap is raised from the volar surface of the forearm, the pattern is marked over an area where a rich venous plexus has been identified. Again, skin, subcutaneous tissue and veins are raised as a unit. Once the flap has been harvested the donor site is either closed primarily or skin-grafted.

CLINICAL EXPERIENCE:

During the period from 1983 to 1986, 25 venous flaps have been performed in 24 patients; these were 19 males and 5 females with a mean age of 32.9. Ten venous flaps were made primarily for soft-tissue coverage with restoration of the venous system for emergency finger replantation or revascularization. Thirteen were performed secondarily as a salvage procedure for replanted digits with venous congestion. Two flaps were done electively for small soft-tissue defects of the hand. Nineteen flaps were harvested from the dorsum of an uninjured finger, four from the volar surface of the forearm, one from the dorsum of the foot, and one from the ulnar aspect of the hand. Six of the 25 flaps were arterialized.

In the 24 patients reviewed, there were 20 successful flaps and five failures. The average age of the patients in each of these two groups was not statistically different. There were also no differences in the patients' medical history, including tobacco habits or medications associated with increased thrombotic risk.

Of the flaps which were successful, 16 were from the dorsum of an uninjured finger, three from the forearm, and one from the dorsum of the foot. Donor sites for flaps which failed included two from the dorsum of an uninjured finger, two from the volar forearm, and one from the ulnar aspect of the hand. The size of the flap had a notable effect on the success rate, since 50% of forearm flaps averaging 12.5 cm^2 failed, compared to an 88% success rate for dorsal finger flaps averaging 6.3 cm^2 in size. In evaluating the overall size of the successful flaps versus the failed flaps, successful flaps averaged 4.6 ± 3.0 cm^2 compared to failed flaps which averaged 9.1 ± 6.9 cm^2 in size. This comparison demonstrated a significance of $P < 0.03$ for smaller flaps favouring better results.

Six of the 25 flaps were arterialized; two-thirds of these survived and one-third failed. There was no statistical benefit to arterialization, although this is a small number for comparison and a more significant trend may be obvious when more patients are added to this series.

Indications for use of the flap did not appear to predetermine the fate of the flap in traumatic cases. Venous flaps used for primary soft-tissue

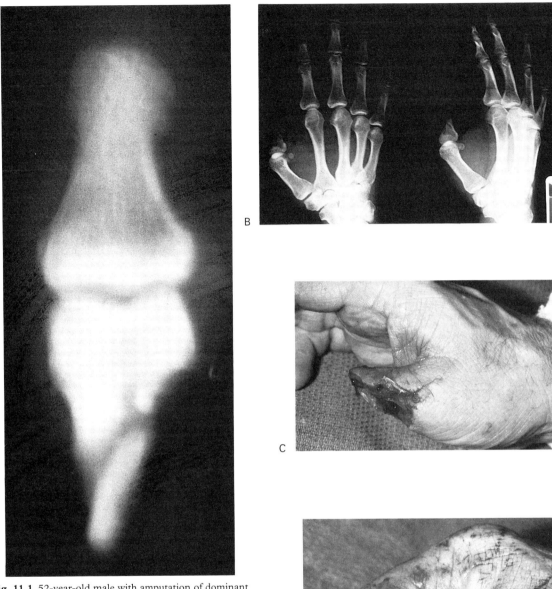

A

B

C

Fig. 11.1 52-year-old male with amputation of dominant thumb through proximal phalanx. **A** AP radiograph of amputated thumb. **B** Radiograph of injured hand. **C** The patient at presentation had a soft-tissue defect along the radial aspect of the proximal phalanx of the thumb.

Fig. 11.2 After bone and soft-tissue reconstruction, a dorsal soft-tissue defect was present over the proximal phalanx. The proximal and distal dorsal veins were isolated and identified for preparation for the venous flap.

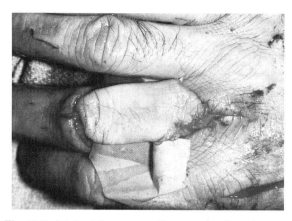

Fig. 11.3 A 1.5 × 4.0 cm venous flap was taken from the dorsum of the middle finger proximal phalanx.

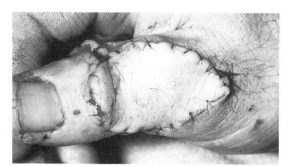

Fig. 11.4 Three proximal and three distal vein-to-vein anastomoses were performed, and the flap was sutured loosely into position.

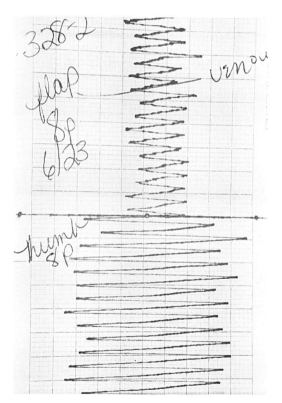

Fig. 11.5 Photoplethysmography (PPG) recording of the replanted thumb and venous flap vascularity.

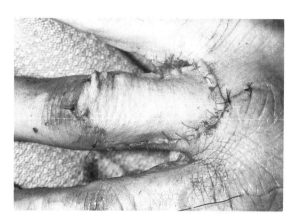

Fig. 11.6 A full-thickness skin graft was used to cover the donor defect.

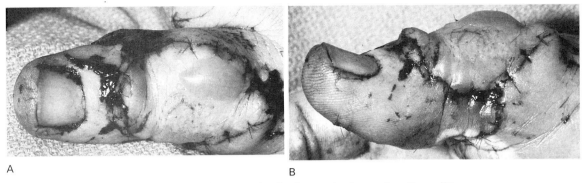

A   B

Fig. 11.7A, B Two days after replantation, the venous free flap has good colour and capillary refill.

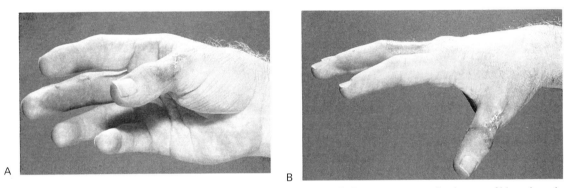

A   B

Fig. 11.8A, B Three months after replantation the patient has good soft-tissue coverage on the dorsum of his replanted thumb.

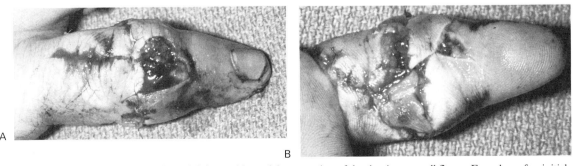

A   B

Fig. 11.9A, B 24-year-old male with crush injury, with partial amputation of the dominant small finger. Four days after initial revascularization with bone, tendon and neurovascular reconstruction, his post-operative course was compromised by persistent venous congestion.

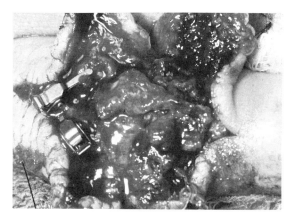

Fig. 11.10 The dorsal veins were found to be thrombosed. The veins and soft tissue were debrided, and the dorsal veins with their thrombosed sections excised were identified and prepared for grafting.

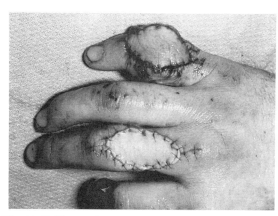

Fig. 11.12 Three vein-to-vein anastomoses were performed distally, with two vein-to-vein anastomoses proximally. The flap provided excellent coverage of the defect. The donor site was grafted was grafted with a full-thickness skin graft from the groin.

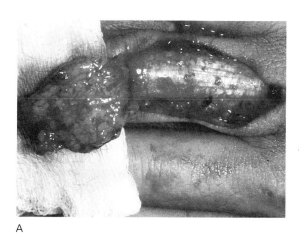

A

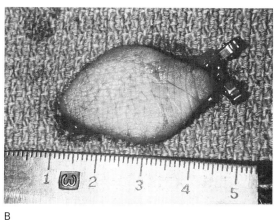

B

Fig. 11.11A, B A 2.0 × 3.5 cm venous flap was taken from the dorsum of the middle finger.

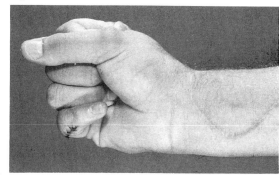

A

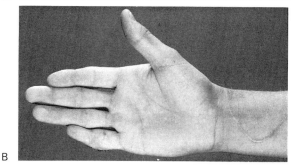

B

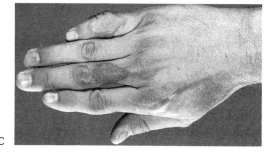

C

Fig. 11.13A, B, C Nine months postoperatively the patient has a good cosmetic and functional result.

defect coverage in replanted or revascularized digits had a 20% failure rate. Flaps used for salvage of a venous congested replanted digit failed in 25% of cases. Elective venous flap coverage of a defect had a 100% success rate.

Of the five venous flaps which failed, four were attributed to lack of inflow due either to anastomotic occlusion or secondary to failed revascularization of the digit. One venous flap failed due to continued venous congestion.

The venous flaps used frequently in this study provide a simple method for the reestablishment of a disrupted or thrombosed venous outflow, while providing skin coverage in one step. This application itself merits the use of this flap, because of its advantages over the use of vein grafts covered with split- or full-thickness skin. Illustrative cases are shown in Figs 11.1–11.13.

DISCUSSION

Over the last 3 years, survival of cutaneous free flaps based only on the venous circulation has been achieved. The success rate of 74% presented in our clinical observations is inferior to the 96% overall success rate with the more extensively applied arteriovenous free flaps. However, there are certain clinical situations in which arteriovenous free flaps or full-thickness skin grafts are not as amenable for soft-tissue coverage. Venous flaps provide full-thickness skin coverage with accompanying vein grafts. Using a venous flap for the indications described provides an easy method of harvesting vein grafts with minimal damage to the veins from dissection, while simultaneously obtaining a full-thickness skin graft. Donor sites for venous flaps are more abundant than for arteriovenous free flaps. The dissection of venous flaps is also less tedious than for arteriovenous flaps. Therefore, if the success rate of venous flaps continues to approach that of arteriovenous free flaps, venous flaps will provide a favourable alternative in various applications.

The physiology of the venous nutrient circulation is not fully understood, and experimental studies must be pursued to clarify this matter. The optimum ratio of vein plexuses and anastomoses per surface area of flap, and the advantages of adding arterial inflow to a venous flap, need to be investigated further.

The authors' clinical experience showing a 74% success rate for venous flaps compares with a 40% complete survival rate of venous flaps for similar indications in the small series of Honda et al (1984). Size is the only statistically significant factor affecting the outcome of the flap. Venous flaps averaging 5 cm^2 in surface area did notably better than flaps averaging approximately 10 cm^2. The other question proposed is whether or not the success rate for the smaller flaps is due to a higher concentration of venous plexuses indigenous to the donor site, with the dorsal finger having a greater concentration of veins per area than the volar forearm. Our series of five forearm venous flaps is not large enough to make any significant statement. Yoshimura et al (1987) reported a series of 12 distal volar forearm arterialized venous flaps, averaging 4–10 cm^2, which had a 100% survival rate. Further clinical studies will clarify the questions of maximum size and the benefits or disadvantages of arterialization.

Our experimental and clinical experience has clarified some of the advantages and disadvantages associated with use of the venous flap. Advantages of the venous flap are:

1. The dissection required to raise a venous flap is less tedious than raising an arteriovenous free flap.
2. The venous flap is less bulky than an arteriovenous free flap.
3. Venous or arterial reconstruction can be performed with the venous flap providing the vein graft for the segmental vascular defect.
4. The venous flap provides full-thickness skin coverage to the area, with better appearance and function than a split-thickness skin graft.
5. A small venous flap can be harvested with no disruption of the arterial supply at the donor site and minimal complications of closure or coverage of the donor site.

The disadvantages of the venous flap are that it is less reliable than an arteriovenous free flap, the circulation is relatively poor when only venous anastomoses are performed, and it appears to be inadequate for coverage of a large area. With more understanding of the venous circulation and more experience with acquired technical skills, venous flaps may become a more reliable alternative for soft-tissue defect coverage, and the clinical applications will probably increase above and beyond the indications reviewed in this chapter.

REFERENCES

Baek S M, Weinberg H, Song R Y et al 1985 Experimental studies in the survival of venous island flaps without arterial inflow. Plastic and Reconstructive Surgery 75: 88–95

Carrel A, Guthrie C 1906 The reversal of circulation in a limb. Annals of Surgery 43: 203–215

Honda T, Nomura S, Yamauchi S et al 1984 The possible application of a composite skin and subcutaneous vein graft in the replantation of amputated digits. British Journal of Plastic Surgery 37: 607–612

Ji S Y, Chia S L, Cheng H H 1984 Free transplantation of venous network pattern skin flap : an experimental study in rabbits. Microsurgery 5: 151–159

Mundy J, Panje W 1984 Creation of free flaps by arterialization of the venous system. Archives of Otolaryngology 110: 221–223

Nakayama Y, Soeda S, Kasai Y 1981 Flaps nourished by arterial inflow through the venous system: an experimental investigation. Plastic and Reconstructive Surgery 67: 328–334

Tsai T, Matiko J, Breidenbach W, Kutz J 1987 Venous flaps in digital revascularization and replantation. Journal of Reconstructive Microsurgery 3: 113–119

Yoshimura M, Shimada T, Imura S et al 1987 The venous skin graft method for repairing skin defects of the fingers. Plastic and Reconstructive Surgery 79: 243–250

12 Tissue expansion in the upper limb

HISTORY

The expansion principle is in evidence all around us. The very nature of normal growth is almost entirely a demonstration of expansion, the expanding force being provided in the trunk and limbs by growing bones. Pregnancy, normal breast development, tumours and obesity all demonstrate the ability of the body to cope with increasing volume by producing more healthy skin. The principle has been in use in surgery for many years. For example, serial excision provides increased skin tension which is the expanding force creating new skin to allow the next excision. Expandable implants provide a means of controlling this expansion force, and have been in use for a relatively short time. The interested reader is referred to the Further Reading section for details of the history of expansion.

INDICATIONS AND GENERAL PRINCIPLES

The need for 'like' skin

The wide variety of reconstructive techniques now available provides the ability to cover practically any skin defect. This skin cover is always provided at a price which may be either scarring at the primary defect site or donor site (cosmetic and/or functional price), or cosmetic and/or functional problems due to the use of skin with characteristics different from the skin it is replacing. The latter problem most commonly results from the use of a skin flap whose bulk of subcutaneous tissue is more appropriate to, for example, a trunk

site, but there are often additional problems of skin match in terms of skin elasticity, colour, hair growth and sensibility. The expansion of healthy skin adjacent to the defect creates extra skin of appropriately similar characteristics, which can be utilized with relatively little scarring.

Time factor

One main limiting factor in skin expansion is the availability of time to expand. The technique is in general inappropriate for the primary management of traumatic skin defects, but planned excisions or secondary reconstructions lend themselves readily to expansion reconstruction. The ISLE (intraoperative sustained limited expansion) technique of Sasaki uses immediate expansion to take maximum advantage of skin elasticity and 'creep', but does not provide new skin (Sasaki 1987). The maximum speed of expansion depends on several factors:

1. *Site* An area with little slack skin normally requires slower expansion than other sites, but thinner skin with little subcutaneous tissue does expand quite readily (Case 6). If there are scars in the skin to be expanded, they will limit the expansion; scarred areas are therefore better avoided if possible. Previously degloved areas are particularly prone to problems when expanded and should rarely be considered.

2. *Pressure* If the pressure within the expander is increased rapidly by a fast injection, pain is more likely than with the same volume injected slowly. The amount injected at each clinic visit should be limited by the patient's symptoms and by the cap-

illary return of the overlying skin. Most patients report that the tension within the area reduces markedly in the first 48 hours after injection, and some work has been carried out on repeated injections at such intervals. The risks of this rapid expansion are those of tissue necrosis, with damage to other structures or exposure of the implant. This could be of particular significance if the underlying tissues include blood vessels or nerves. Recent evidence suggests that capsule formation around the implant is less likely if the expansion is completed in a relatively short time, thus favouring frequent injections. A continuous infusion controlled by a constant pressure head may provide an optimal answer in terms of speed of expansion.

3. *Convenience* The expansion timetable should be kept as flexible as possible. Sometimes frequent clinic visits may be precluded by distance, and a longer term of expansion may be more acceptable. Injections may be delegated to other physicians provided they understand the aims and potential problems. Some patients may be able to carry out their own injections. Others may have a limited hospital stay during which all the work must be completed.

Tolerance of temporary disfigurement

The expander itself may produce functional limitations from its sheer bulk, or cosmetic disfigurement that is unacceptable. An approximate timetable and a realistic explanation of the appearance and possible problems should be discussed with the patient before an expander is inserted.

EXPANDER DESIGN

Expanders are available in a very wide range of shapes and sizes. Most of the shapes possible have been made using 'Mandrills' or moulds. Once this mould has been made it is available for making as many expanders as required. There are structural variations, but all expanders are made of a silicone polymer material, which is usually collapsed in folds when the expander is empty. Expansion is initially an unfolding and filling of the 'bag', fol-

lowed by a stretching of the wall. This stretching property varies with different makes of implant.

Some expanders have a semirigid base which theoretically produces a more vertical expansion of the expander from this base. If these are used on a convex surface there is a potential problem with the edge of the reinforced base: as the expansion proceeds, the base, which initially conforms to the convexity, becomes flatter (more tangential to the convexity) and its edge can cause pressure problems on the skin.

A recent development is an expander which is semirigid with an elastic 'patch' in the top surface. The expander is completely flat when empty and the elastic patch expands along predictable lines. The elasticity of the patch can be varied in design to give eccentric expansion if required. At present these suffer from the same drawbacks as the other semirigid base expanders, plus the additional problem of the pressure which may be exerted by the thick reinforced rim of these prostheses.

Those expanders with symmetrical structure provide radial as well as vertical expansion. The shape of the expander is chosen to make the best use of available skin, and to provide a particular shape of extra skin to suit the reconstruction.

INJECTION PORT DESIGN

The self-sealing implantable injection port is now available in a variety of sizes and shapes to cause minimal cosmetic and functional problems, and to aid removal. Alternatively the tubing from the expander can be led through a tunnel and out through the skin, to be used without injecting the patient. This has the potential problem of sepsis via the tube track, but this possibility is reduced if a Dacron cuff is incorporated at the site of exit through the skin, or by increasing the distance between implant and tube exit site. Some expanders are also available with an integral expansion port which has an impenetrable back plate. These can cause difficulties if placed beneath thin skin such as at the wrist, as the port has a raised rim which can cause local pressure problems and the additional problem from the small dead space that exists within the rim of the injection port (Fig. 12.6A).

COSTS

Re-use of expanders

When the expander is removed and the skin utilized, the expander may be emptied and replaced in order to repeat the expansion in situations where a larger area of skin is required. This has been found useful in the piecemeal removal of large benign skin lesions such as giant hairy naevi. The injection ports of earlier models were more limited in the number of times they could be pierced without leaking. If leaks are a potential problem with reuse, the injection port can be replaced at the second stage.

Some surgeons regularly save removed expanders, resterilizing and using them for other patients. The argument against this is the possible introduction of infection or the antigenicity of small particles of skin introduced by the injections into the injection port. Adequate sterilization procedures should prevent the infection problem; changing the injection port removes the antigenic problem. The remaining problem of a higher leakage rate from the expander (or injection port if it is reused) is one for the individual surgeon to decide upon. In a state health system it may be justified to accept the increased risk of leakage if the reuse of the expander allows a patient to be treated who would otherwise be denied this technique. However, more hospitals are now becoming conscious of the potential medicolegal hazards of this approach and specifically forbid this practice.

PLANNING

The aim is to introduce the expander into the desired site without additional scars wherever possible. Sasaki has stressed the principle of using an access wound that lies radially, to minimize the chances of wound dehiscence. In practice the author has not had difficulties with tangential or marginal wounds, provided they lie just outside the edge of the expander, and the incision should be made through good skin adjacent to the scarring to be replaced. The means of utilization of the skin should be established in advance. In many instances the skin will be simply advanced after

expansion; however, this is not efficient. Efficiency is increased by the use of the 'croissant', a curved design of expander. An alternative is a transposition flap from within the expanded skin: the base of the flap advances as the secondary defect closes, and provides a more efficient utilization of the expanded skin (Godfrey 1984, 1987).

Syndactyly has been treated with the help of skin expansion (Fenton 1987, Van Beek & Adson 1987, Watson & Kay 1989, personal communication). The author does not feel that this technique has sufficient advantage over full-thickness skin grafts to justify the additional surgery and multiple clinic visits for the injections.

Although flap skin for the digit is often required, expansion within the digit is rarely used, as the requirement is most often immediate. There is a place for expansion in secondary flap provision where avoidance of the scarring of local or cross-finger flaps, or of the complexity of microsurgical techniques, is desired. Van Beek and Adson (1987) reported using a custom expander in a digit tip to create sufficient skin to allow insertion of a bone graft and achieve 1 cm of useful length.

Abdominal or groin flaps may be expanded in advance to provide large areas of skin for arm cover. This minimizes the trunk defect.

PROBLEMS

Children

Frequent injections may be upsetting for a child and an exteriorized injection port may at times be preferable. Conversely children are more likely to interfere with the exteriorized tube or port and the pain of injections may be ameliorated by the use of topical anaesthesia such as EMLA cream.

Infection

True infection is very unusual, provided the overlying skin remains intact and the injection technique is sterile. Contamination of the implant at insertion increases the risk of marked capsule formation, which will limit the expansion but may still allow sufficient expansion to be achieved with antibiotic control. After removal of the expander

Illustration cases

Case 1 Release of burn-scarred adducted shoulder (Figs 12.1A–12.1E).

This 46-year-old diabetic man had severely limited abduction of the right shoulder 8 months after a full-thickness burn was grafted. The simple expansion provided a healthy flap to break up the tethered band of scar and allow recovery of normal shoulder movement. A common feature of expansion adjacent to an ulcerated area is that the ulcer often heals during the expansion, partly as a result of increased vascularity and partly by the reduction of mobility and stress that the expansion produces.

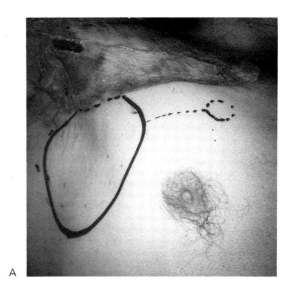

A

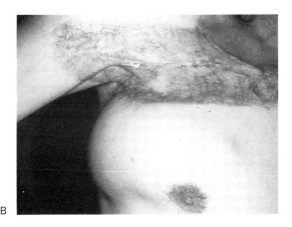

B

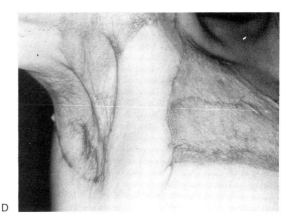

D

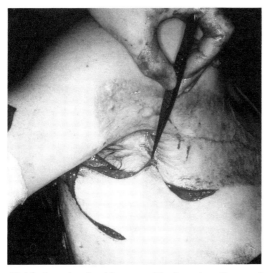

C

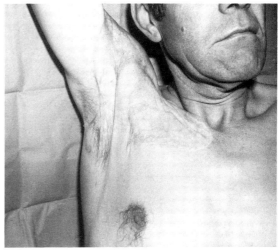

E

Fig. 12.1A Anterior shoulder scar with ulceration. Proposed expander site outlined. **B** Expansion almost complete. Ulcer healed. **C** Expander removed. Transposition/advancement flap incised. **D** One month after division/release of scar and flap inset. Abduction 90°. **E** Two months later. Full abduction.

Case 2 Provision of durable cover for shoulder joint (Figs 12.2A–12.2D).

This self-employed man suffered a traumatic amputation of his left arm. He was eager to return to work but was unable to tolerate the necessary prosthesis because of its pressure on unstable grafted skin at the injury site. Expansion provided healthy flap skin which enabled him to use the prosthesis and return to work.

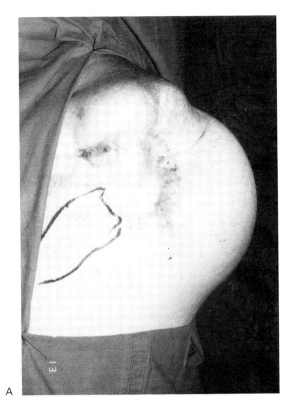

A

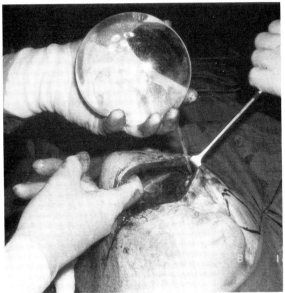

B

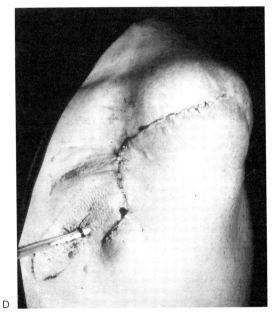

D

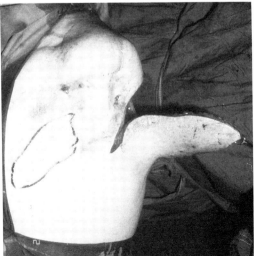

C

Fig. 12.2A Lateral view of left arm avulsion scar. Axillary hair-bearing area outlined. Expander in scapular area. **B** Expander removal viewed from above shoulder. **C** Flap raised (viewed as in A). **D** Flap transposed and advanced across glenoid area after excision of scarred skin.

Case 3 Thigh transposition/advancement flap for maximum efficiency (Figs 12.3A–12.3C).

This case demonstrates maximum skin utilization from a spherical expander in the limbs.

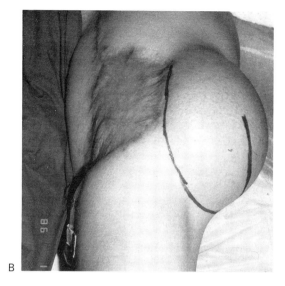

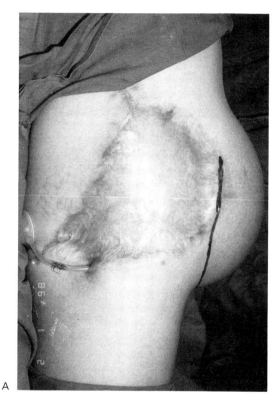

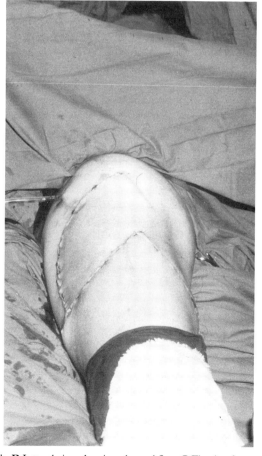

Fig. 12.3A Graft and scar of proximal thigh. Expander in lateral thigh. **B** Lateral view showing planned flap. **C** Flap in after scar excision and direct closure of donor site.

Case 4 Serial reexpansion of skin to remove a giant pigmented naevus (Figs 12.4A–12.4H).

The case shown is of a giant hairy naevus involving much of the right lower limb. The principles and practice are the same as in the upper limb. On completion of the first operation to use the expanded skin flap, the expander was deflated and reinserted under the newly expanded skin. The programme of expansion was then repeated three times with no apparent limitation from using already expanded skin.

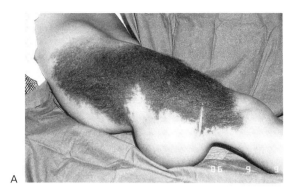

A

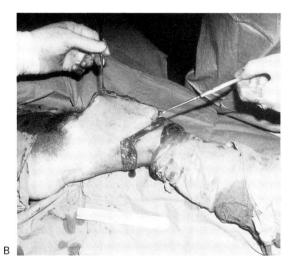

B

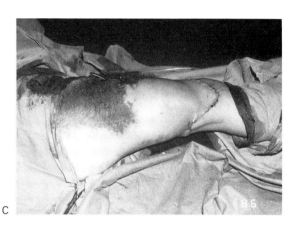

C

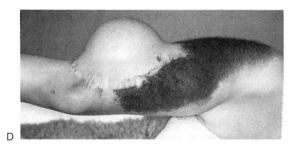

D

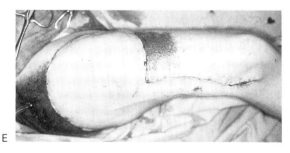

E

Fig. 12.4A Giant pigmented naevus – iliac crest to knee. First expander above popliteal fossa. **B** Flap advanced and transposed after removing first expander and excising distal naevus. **C** Second expander placed beneath the flap at same procedure as B. **D** Second expansion complete. **E** Second flap transposed and advanced. Third expander placed beneath flap. **F** Third expansion complete. **G** Third flap procedure. Fourth expander placed beneath flap. **H** After healing of fourth expansion flap procedure. Scar revisions planned for 1 year.

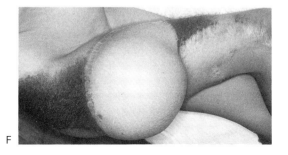

F

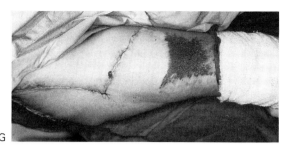

G

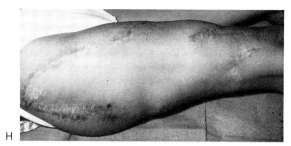

H

Case 5 Lift-off technique to remove large naevi/tattoos (Figs 12.5A–12.5C).

This case shows the lift-off technique applied to a congenital pigmented naevus occupying 45% of the wrist circumference. Expansion of the naevus itself was limited by the prior insertion of an encircling nylon suture within the dermis of the naevus margin (Godfrey 1984).

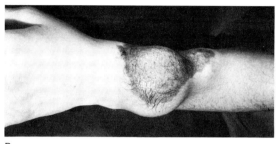

B

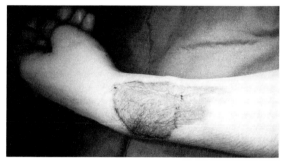

A

Fig. 12.5A Expander inserted beneath naevus. Dermal nylon encircling suture in place. **B** Expansion almost complete beneath naevus of wrist. **C** After excision of 80% of naevus.

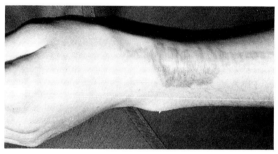

C

Case 6 Distal volar wrist expansion to cover nerve reconstruction (Figs 12.6A, B).

This young woman lost volar ulnar wrist skin together with 4 cm of ulnar nerve in a road traffic accident. She was referred for repair of the nerve. Skin cover was provided by expansion of adjacent skin. The expander was one with a clumsy, thick integral injection port which produced small areas of pressure necrosis, and further complicated matters because of the dead space in the well of the port. The skin was utilized successfully to cover the nerve grafts, but this bulky form of integral injection port should be avoided in such areas.

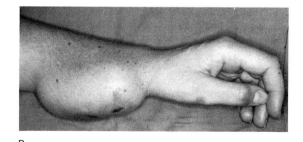

B

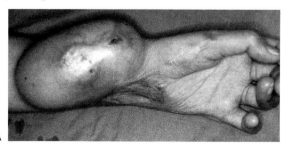

A

Fig. 12.6A Expansion complete across volar wrist. Adjacent scarred graft overlies ulnar nerve defect. The resultant flap was transposed/advanced at the time of nerve graft for reconstruction of the ulnar nerve. **B** Lateral view of expansion.

Case 7 Skin augmentation to facilitate digital transfer (Figs 12.7A–12.7F).

This boy lost the thumb and index rays completely and only the three ulnar metacarpals were salvaged following a firework accident. The case demonstrates the provision of sufficient skin by expansion of adjacent areas to cover the toe transfer. The head of the transferred metatarsal was fixed to the trapezium.

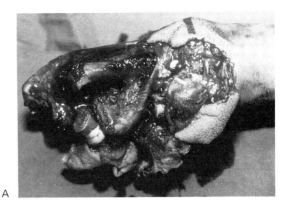

A

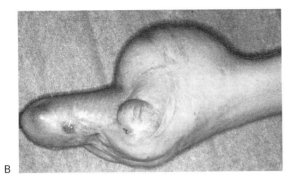

B

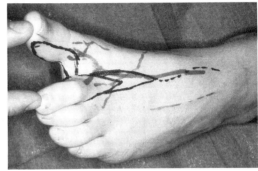

C

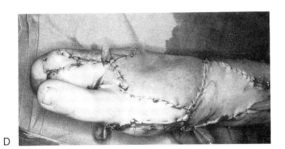

D

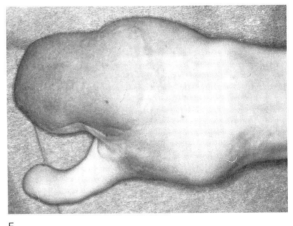

E

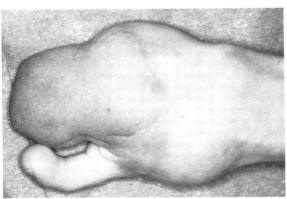

F

Fig. 12.7A Firework explosion injury of right hand. **B** Expansion of dorsal wrist skin under way. **C** Planned transfer of second toe and adjacent innervated skin. **D** Toe + sensate skin transfer completed utilizing transposition/advancement of expanded skin to cover the dorsal transfer defect. **E, F** Functional span of reconstruction.

the infection usually clears rapidly. There is commonly a phase of redness of the expanding skin, which may simulate infection. This is due to an increased vascularity stimulated by the expansion force and is not accompanied by additional swelling or pain. This redness subsides after removal of the expander and utilization of the skin. In negroid skin hyperpigmentation may follow this redness and takes much longer to resolve.

Necrosis

This should be foreseen and forestalled by removing fluid from the expander and reducing the pressure. At times a fold of the implant wall may form a localized pressure point, and in this case input of additional fluid to unfold the wall may overcome the problem. Two cases have been seen in which the overlying skin was perfectly viable, but the capsule and deeper tissues on the deep surface of the implant were partly necrosed. If there is partial necrosis over the injection port, this need not halt expansion provided sepsis can be prevented, or at least controlled.

Pain

Pain at injection time is related to pressure, and is more likely if the injection is given too rapidly or if too much is given. The injection of 5–10 ml of 1%

lignocaine into the implant has been found helpful by some when pain appears to be unrelated to an excessive expansion force.

Leakage

Leakage should be tested for in each implant prior to insertion. Skin closure over the expander must be carried out with due care, as any pinpricks in the implant or tubing render it useless. The lie of the tubing in relation to the injection port should also be carefully controlled and noted, as subsequent injections may miss the injection port and could puncture the tubing. The tubing should never cross over the injection port. The injection port should be placed away from the expander so that there is no risk of puncturing the implant during injections. It may be necessary to insert a suture at the initial operation to ensure that the injection port does not slip into the main cavity with the expander. Sometimes the injection port may flip over and become inaccessible if the pocket made for it is too large.

Limitation of joint movement

The effect of splinting of a joint by an adjacent expander must be carefully assessed in advance, in order to prevent problems of function which may occur from prolonged limitation of movement.

REFERENCES AND FURTHER READING

Argenta L C, Watanabe M J, Grabb W C, Newmann M H 1981 Soft tissue expander in head and neck surgery. A new method of reconstruction. Plastic Surgery Forum 4

Austad E D, Rose G L 1982 A self-inflating implant for donor tissue augmentation. Plastic and Reconstructive Surgery 70: 588–593

Cherry G, Austad E, Pasyk K et at 1983 Increased survival of random pattern skin flaps elevated in controlled, expanded skin. Plastic and Reconstructive Surgery 72: 680–685

Fenton O 1987 Expansion in the treatment of syndactyly. Presented at the Winter Meeting of the British Association of Plastic Surgeons (unpublished)

Francis A J, Marks R 1977 Skin stretching and epidermopoeisis. British Journal of Experimental Pathology 58: 35

Godfrey A M 1984 Extremity reconstruction. Presented at the Oxford Symposium on Tissue Expansion in Reconstructive Surgery, February 1984. (unpublished)

Godfrey A M 1987, Efficient utilisation of expanded skin.

Presented at the Tissue Expansion Symposia, Harrogate 1987 & Gleneagles 1988. (unpublished)

Lapin R, Daniel D, Hutchins H, Justice G 1980 Primary breast reconstruction followed mastectomy using a skin-expander prosthesis. Breast 6: 20

Neumann G 1957 The expansion of an area of skin by progressive distension of a subcutaneous balloon. Plastic and Reconstructive Surgery 19: 124–130

Radovan C 1976 Adjacent flap development using expandable silastic implants. American Society of Plastic & Reconstructive Surgery, Forum, Boston, Mass.

Radovan C 1982 Breast reconstruction after mastectomy using the temporary expander. Plastic and Reconstructive Surgery 69: 2

Sasaki G H 1987 Intraoperative sustained limited expansion (ISLE) as an immediate reconstructive technique. In: Tissue expansion. Clinics in Plastic Surgery, W B Saunders, Philadelphia

Van Beek A L, Adson M H 1987 Tissue expansion in the upper extremity. In: Tissue expansion, Clinics in Plastic Surgery. W B Saunders, Philadelphia

John Colville

13 The management of skin loss on the dorsum of the hand and finger

The many differing situations associated with trauma to the dorsum of the hand, and the many other factors influencing treatment, demand a knowledge of the basic anatomical and physiological features of the area. With such an understanding, the solution to any particular problem should be capable of rationalization. This is preferable to a prescribed treatment for a given situation or set of circumstances, and while later in this chapter a few conditions and their treatment are referred to, this is only because they do not conform to the usual treatment guidelines. The basic approach to the management of problems in this area does not require the memorizing of details to nearly the same extent as would be required by reference to precise injuries and their corresponding treatment. This approach should be capable of application and adaptation to meet most situations, encourage an open-minded attitude towards each injury encountered, and is conducive to the modification of techniques and methods of managemant leading to improved hand care.

SKIN MOBILITY

The skin on the dorsum of the hand is unique in having a degree of mobility specialized to meet the requirements of flexion and extension and a certain amount of shearing, without disruption. The palmar skin follows in a reciprocal fashion, but does so mainly by folding and unfolding between attachments, represented by crease lines. On the palm there is relatively little stretch.

The dorsal skin, from a resting position with the hand outstretched, allows flexion by a combination of skin stretch over the metacarpal area and an unfolding of the skin wrinkles over the proximal interphalangeal (PIP) joints. The skin wrinkling gradually extends more proximally to the metacarpal area in the elderly, whose skin elasticity is progressively reduced. To accommodate these features of wrinkling and elasticity, it follows that dorsal skin must be only loosely attached to the structures it covers, and for this reason is susceptible to shearing forces which can quite readily detach the skin at a subdermal fat level. The apparent surplus of skin on the dorsum, seen with the hand in the extended position, is completely taken up by flexion. The implications of this fact affect two different types of clinical situation.

Where graft replacement of skin of the dorsum of the fingers and the hand is undertaken, this must *not* be done with the metacarpophalangeal (MP) or PIP joints in the extended position, otherwise insufficient skin will be inserted into the defect to allow full flexion. Full flexion of the MP joints and partial flexion of the PIP joints is necessary. If extension of the PIP joint is required for other reasons, this can be adjusted in 5 days, when the graft should have become vascularized.

Where the excision of damaged skin is necessary, the apparent surplus of skin should not tempt the surgeon into primary closure of a defect, unless this can be achieved fairly easily and still allow reasonable finger flexion after wound closure.

Associated with this attachment of skin there are relatively few deep perforating vessels supplying arterial blood, and most of the skin on the dorsum of the hand is dependent on an intrinsic form of skin circulation derived more proximally. This type of blood supply is more easily compromised by tension across the suture lines that elsewhere would have no significant effect. These considerations are well borne out by the delay in wound healing seen in relatively small defects which have been inadvisably sutured, or where damage to traumatized skin is compounded by the added trauma of suture under tension. A further exacerbating effect associated with loose skin attachment is the tendency to allow swelling. The loose subdermal areolar space readily accommodates oedema fluid, and this can add to the difficulties associated with wound closure.

The special mobility of the dorsal skin, which advances distally over the flexing joints, must be reproduced in any alternative form of skin cover. A graft or flap must be equally mobile. This may determine their boundary lines so that these do not adhere to a fixed point, or become shortened or contracted. In the latter case it may be necessary to sacrifice normal dorsal skin, particularly on the dorsum of the fingers, so that the margin of a flap or graft may be close to the midaxial line. For split-skin grafts to reproduce the normal dorsal skin mobility it is mandatory that a guaranteed full take of skin is achieved, and this can only be so if all the factors governing the take of skin – namely, fixation, bed-vascularity and complete haemostasis – are guaranteed. The various features of the loosely attached dorsal skin, which make this in many respects more vulnerable than skin elsewhere, provide one major redeeming feature: consequent upon removal of this skin at subdermal level, the bed provides a recipient area for a free thick split graft that can take readily and provide an adhesion-free durable alternative skin cover, which can come close to resembling normal skin.

NERVE SUPPLY

The nerve supply to the dorsum of the hand and fingers is mainly from the terminal branches of the radial nerve, with contributions from the ulnar and median nerves. Loss of sensation is significant, but not too serious from a functional point of view. There will be a permanent disconcerting absence of sensation in a variable area, represented by the nerve distribution, with a marginal zone of sensation whose quality is diminished. Occasionally the radial nerve supply to the thumb encroaches on the volar aspect of the distal pulp. Damage to this might slightly affect the quality of sensation at the sides of the pulp, but not sufficiently to affect dexterity requiring sensory discrimination.

The radial nerve also seems particularly prone to developing pathological neuromata of its branches if these are divided or traumatized, and this may have a much more serious clinical effect than the corresponding sensory loss. The radial nerve branches are easy to repair at the wrist level, and not too difficult as far as the MP joint level. Division should be rectified by a primary repair, not only to restore sensation but equally to avoid the occasional quite troublesome neuroma that can follow division.

BLOOD SUPPLY

The blood supply to the dorsum is mainly on a longitudinal basis via the metacarpal arteries. These arise from the dorsal carpal arch, which receives contributions mainly from the radial artery, the dorsal interosseous artery and the terminal branch of the volar interosseous artery. The ulnar artery also contributes to the dorsal blood supply in about 30% of cases (Coleman & Anson 1961). The dorsum of the lower forearm and adjacent carpal area is supplied from the dorsal carpal network of vessels, which is distributed distally in the form of well-defined metacarpal arteries on the dorsal aspect of the interosseous muscles. The first dorsal metacarpal artery is usually present (89% of cases) but is frequently quite a small vessel. The second metacarpal artery is usually a little larger and supplies skin as far as the dorsum of the proximal interphalangeal (IP) joint. In Coleman and Anson's dissections of 75 specimens this vessel was present in 98.7%. The third metacarpal artery, of equal size and supplying the same extent of skin, was found in 98%, and the fourth metacarpal artery in 81%. This metacarpal artery, invariably arising from the termination of the ulnar artery, may not supply skin as far distally as the other metacarpal arteries. The dorsal metacarpal arteries also usually have a deep communication with the volar metacarpal arteries at the distal metacarpal level.

The territory supplied by these vessels is becoming increasingly recognized with the utilization of small axial flaps taken from the dorsum of the MP joint and proximal phalanx areas. Beyond the MP joint the dorsal digital branches from the digital arteries reinforce the true dorsal supply, and provide the main arterial supply to the distal two-thirds of the dorsum of the finger. Clinical observations would suggest that the proximal part of the metacarpal area and the carpal skin depends on a random pattern of blood supply, and the survival of any part of an isolated skin area cannot be expected to extend much beyond a distance equal to the width of its base in this area.

Since most of the venous drainage of the hand passes proximally through the dorsal veins, these are large but not too numerous. Admittedly one or two may be sacrificed, but care should be exercised in preserving as many as possible. These can be retracted easily in the loose areolar tissue in which they are found, and with the loss of perhaps a few side branches the main dorsal veins can be preserved and this should be done as far as possible. Certainly if there is extensive damage to this area, exploration to establish a surgical diagnosis and undertake repair must not make matters worse by further loss of veins. This applies particularly to roller compression injuries in which there is a crushing component as well as shearing damage to the dorsal skin. In such a situation it is well recognized that swelling is a particularly troublesome and protracted accompaniment to the injury. The sacrifice of any veins in the debridement of such a wound can be seen to exacerbate this problem.

TENDON LAYER

This lies between the deep side of the loose fatty areolar layer, deep to the veins, and includes the investing condensation of deep fascia which forms the dorsal retinacular layer. This is quite thin over the metacarpals and phalanges, where it may be difficult to recognize, but more proximally over the carpus and lower forearm substantial thickening of the fascia condenses to form the extensor compartments. Removal of the superficial investing fascia leaves the tendons covered by paratenon only, and it is a matter of priority that this must be covered immediately to preserve its integrity. In the short term this is done by ensuring that some form of moist cover is applied as soon as the wound is inspected. This may be done by taping detached skin flaps back in position, or if this still leaves paratenon exposed, a moist saline dressing will preserve it for some hours. Also, during subsequent surgery in which paratenon is exposed, this must not be allowed to become dry. Removal of the paratenon leaves the tendons exposed and if these are not covered by some form of vascularized tissue as a matter of urgency, they will not survive.

The exact method of providing cover for exposed tendons is determined by a number of factors. The size and location of the defect may allow the transposition of local skin with a safe proximal base to cover a limited area. This flap is raised, as are all resections and underminings of this area, at the fatty areolar plane, leaving a secondary defect whose successful grafting will not to any extent detract from the usefulness of such a flap for a small distal metacarpal or phalangeal defect. The type of injury, however, may determine whether or not a local flap can be considered safe. When damaged, the skin edge may not survive as the distal border of a flap which in elective circumstances would be quite safe, and for that reason in many wounds of the dorsum of the hand a distant flap or free flap is necessary. Quite often the nature of the injury also determines the mode of distant flap cover. Crush injuries, gunshot wounds and other untidy injuries are particularly predisposed to post-traumatic oedema, but this may make the groin flap or any other dependent flap a less than ideal remedy, because of the essential dependency of the hand for 3 weeks, during which time the flap picks up its new blood supply. If a flap is used in such circumstances, then a cross-arm flap is preferable to one attached to the groin. Better still is the reverse radial artery forearm flap, or a distant free flap, in order not to compromise the appearance of the forearm, especially in females.

BONE

The necessity for certain types of fixation may also determine the form of flap cover required. Metacarpal plate fixation might just impart sufficient extra damage to the already injured skin to make this too risky a combination of foreign body, added bulk and uncertain skin survival, and in this situation either the plating is omitted or an alternative and safer form of cover is provided which will allow the safe plating of underlying metacarpal fractures. The much smaller 'miniplates' recently introduced now allow plate fixation in most situations on the back of the hand, but the above reservations about added material must still be considered at all times.

In all these matters the skin cover has priority. No matter how sophisticated and technically expert the repair of bone, tendon or joint, it is more than likely to be for nothing if the overlying skin and soft tissues do not survive. The need for early movement may also make the constraint of an added distant flap unacceptable, and the availability of an increasing variety of free flaps provides a convenient form of repair, allowing whatever movement is indicated.

Perhaps it is unnecessary with today's standard of hand care to refer to the archaic practice of burying the hand under a bridge, or into a pocket, of abdominal skin. This mode of treatment cannot be considered under any circumstances and is in all situations completely contraindicated.

PRINCIPLES OF MANAGEMENT

These can be reduced to the care of the skin and the care of the repaired underlying functional structures as they relate to skin. Skin care begins with an assessment of its viability when damaged. Visually this can be quite misleading, and there is a need to recognize the severity of the situation particularly in hot press burns and crush injuries. Bleeding at the skin edge *may* indicate survival, but care should be exercised to ensure that the so-called bleeding is not simply a venous ooze. Edge bleeding must be active capillary bleeding if survival is to be expected. Inflation of a tourniquet for 5 minutes and observation for reactive hyperaemia will emphasize whatever skin circulation is available, and *may* indicate the distal extent of guaranteed circulation. At this level of doubtful survival, response to pinprick is of no value in determining the skin's vascularity. Avulsed skin is seldom viable for more than 1 cm or so from its undamaged attached proximal edge. Thrombosis of the dermal vessels confirms a definite loss of viability. Intravenous dyes have at times been recommended but their use is not practical. If the skin is damaged beyond survival, or without evidence of circulation, it must be resected back to a level of guaranteed survival. There is nothing worse in this situation than the finding of a resected area of skin successfully grafted, only to find a strip of necrotic skin proximal to this; or to find a flap inserted into a defect one edge of which is completely necrotic, when it would have been quite simple to have resected a further margin of skin without disadvantage. Occasionally there is an area of skin damage whose viability cannot be determined, which from the history of injury and appearance might just survive. In such a situation a trial of survival may succeed, and if so a good deal of extra treatment may be avoided. The edge of the damaged skin is trimmed with a scalpel, removing no more than 1 mm – sutured in place, dressed and immobilized in plaster of Paris in such a position as to relax the tension across the skin junction. This is inspected 48 hours later, when a decision about the skin's viability will be declared by its obvious condition. There is no place for providing a window in the dressings through which the skin may be observed during this period. Frequent observations by different persons in different lights are a waste of time; furthermore the exposure and possible prodding and handling of a surgical wound are not conducive to good wound healing even in healthy skin, and much less so in questionably viable skin. If at 48 hours the skin is dead then it is removed and replaced. The inspection is done under theatre conditions with the provision to proceed with surgery if indicated. There is no place whatsoever for awaiting the separation of a slough except for the smallest defects (less than 10 mm). Slough separation and edge healing should be avoided, since they produce deep scar formation with adhesion of the underlying skin to tendons, and possibly adhesion between tendon and bone. Chronic oedema and eventual conversion of the oedema to scar tissue by its infiltration with fibroblasts is a well-recognized pathological process, which if established cannot be reversed. This frequently follows slow wound healing and accounts for a chronically swollen and indurated back of hand.

Where there is *apparent* wellbeing of the skin initially, it is essential that the patient or his parent is fully informed of the doubtful nature of the skin. The immediate healthy appearance of the skin contrasts sharply with the eventual flap that may be necessary to replace it, and it is essential that this is fully appreciated by all concerned.

Whether to suture loosely with widely spaced sutures or with fine material closely spaced is an old debate which can be directed at the situation pertaining to many dorsal skin injuries. This argument may already have been settled, but the matter may be finalized by reaffirming that, provided skin-edge care is maintained to the highest standard, the insertion of sufficient sutures in sufficient numbers to approximate the skin edges in a position most conducive to capillary bridging and healing by first intention, gives skin the best chance of survival. If drainage is required then this can be attended to by a purpose-designed drain, and not one through the edge of the wound. If a stab drain is inserted, care should also be exercised that this does not penetrate a proximal vein.

Healing by first intention is an absolute requirement, whether applied to skin edge closure, skin grafting or flap cover. Secondary healing is to be avoided, not only because of the delay in healing and mobilization of the hand, but also because of the deep scar formation and its attendant stiffness and restriction of tendon excursion.

THE UNDERLYING TENDONS

Decisions about the provision of skin cover must take into account the condition of the underlying tendons. If these are intact it should be possible, however tattered they may be, to conserve continuity if immediate vascular cover can be provided. Debridement should be confined to picking out particulate debris only. Trimming of loose parts of the tendons is not advised, but rather these should be arranged alongside the intact tendons in such a way as to reinforce those that remain. In tendon injury with severe damage, all of the visible tendon in the wound is probably already avascular and subject to the physiological constraints of a free graft, so there is no point in resecting strands of tendon attached only at one or other end. These should be rearranged in the best available position, and their survival can be expected if they can achieve vascularization. The real difficulty in tendon damage is the associated damage to the structures above (skin) and below (bone), to which they may adhere if there is delay in healing.

Where there is loss of both tendon and skin, split-skin grafting followed by Silastic tendon spacers, and subsequently by tendon grafts have reportedly given excellent functional and cosmetic results (Bevin & Hothem 1978). This method of treatment might be best reserved for the elderly, in whom sophisticated free flaps or attached flaps might be contraindicated.

The standard recommendation and most certain procedure following skin and tendon avulsion is that provided for by a groin or radial forearm flap, under which flat tendon spacers are inserted at the same time. The ends of these Silastic spacers must not coincide with the flap margins, otherwise there is a distinct tendency for the ends of the spacers to erode through the scar between the flap and the normal skin, especially at the distal junction. This is caused by the inherent tendency of the rods to remain straight whilst finger flexion is regained, with the result that the spacers exert pressure on the underside of the scar. For this reason Silastic spacers must extend for 1–2 cm beyond the flap margin, so that on acute flexion their ends impinge on healthy skin.

The dorsalis pedis free flap has been used because of the easily available tendon complement already vascularized on the undersurface of the flap. This is at the price of foot disfigurement, which is too expensive both cosmetically and functionally for a single or even a double extensor tendon loss situation. Where three, and particularly four, tendons are lost – in which case there are no tendons available to provide tendon transfers to the extensor-deficient fingers – the dorsalis pedis flap and an immediate tendon reconstruction should be considered.

BONE DAMAGE

It should be stressed again that internal fixation must not further damage the skin, and that without proper skin cover or its healthy alternative any such intervention is likely to lead to the eventual removal of metal and its replacement by external immobilization, slow bone union, scarred soft tissue and joint stiffness, due to prolonged immobilization and adherent extensor tendons.

If at all possible, extra cover for fractures, and especially those that have been further traumatized by fixation, is essential if the overlying extensor tendons are not to become very densely adherent. This is seen over the distal metacarpal area, and particularly over the dorsum of the proximal phalanges. The introduction of a small flap of fat, or vascularized areolar tissue, sufficient to give a viable separating layer between tendons and bone, can be of benefit. To do this there must be either healthy overlying local skin, or flap cover. If the overlying skin is in any way devitalized this should not be further compromised by the separation of a layer of fat from its undersurface. All the foregoing considerations should provide guidance and direction in the provision of skin cover following injury. A few specialized types of injury merit more detail.

BITES AND SIMILAR INJURIES

Human and animal bites are frequently accompanied by the inoculation of the damaged tissue with saliva, and this can give rise to swelling and stiffness which may be troublesome for many months before settling. The bite wound is at times a simple punctate skin wound, but is frequently accompanied by a torn portion of skin that can be managed differently. The torn part of the wound should be very lightly edge-trimmed with a scalpel, and sutured as for any other wound. The punctate portion, which has been crushed and is probably also inoculated with saliva, more so than the remainder of the wound, should be more liberally debrided and left open. Prophylactic antibiotics, including those that are active against staphylococci and anaerobic bacteria, are recommended from the outset. The hand should be totally immobilized for the first week in a plaster of Paris slab combined with a sling. Following this, increasing periods of release from immobilization are advised, during which the patient recovers active and passive movement. This intermittent rest and exercise regimen continues until the swelling is reasonably under control, and the patient should be warned that this may take some weeks.

Other bites, such as those caused by spiders and insects, are much less common. The injected toxin which is usually responsible for the skin damage or skin loss should be identified by reference to the animal producing the injury. In some instances the damaged skin is best excised and grafted, and advice regarding the management of such injuries should always be sought from a surgeon conversant with this type of injury, in whichever geographical area this occurs.

OIL AND PAINT INJECTION INJURIES

These seldom affect the dorsum of the hand primarily, but if so, they are much more favourably treated than elsewhere. The injection of an irritant may evoke a considerable amount of reaction but this is usually confined to the subcutaneous tissue. This is relatively easily 'debrided' and should be tackled energetically. The persistence of such an irritant in a subcutaneous space will lead to reactive swelling and adjacent joint stiffness. This will become irreversibly established if one waits until the underlying necrotic tissue sloughs out. It is preferable to excise this initially, removing all doubtful tissue and applying a graft to the back of the hand, using split skin as an initial dressing. If this does not take, or if more debridement is necessary, the grafting is repeated until skin cover is finally achieved. Again it must be emphasized that the separation of a slough on the back of the hand should not be awaited, but the tissue that would give rise to slough should be removed and the defect repaired.

The injection injury on the palmar aspect of the hand may involve the back of the hand, but seldom results in the loss of skin cover; instead it may cause secondary oedema which, like all other sources of oedema in this area, is liable to become replaced by scar tissue if allowed to persist for too long.

IATROGENIC INJURY

Injury of the dorsum of the hand associated with the delivery of an irritant substance which may leak or be delivered extravenously is also an occasional problem, particularly in neonatal and cardiac units. A problem usually arises when there is an attempted delivery of a hypertonic or irritant solution into collapsed veins in extenuating circumstances. The injury should be recognized and referred to someone who is competent in the management of this as soon as the patient has survived sufficiently to make treatment possible. The damage is proportional to the amount of substance deposited in the subcutaneous tissue, and this must be quite frankly discussed with whoever had the information about the concentration and volume of substance in question.

If seen within an hour or so of the injury, the correct management is a small incision through which the products of the damaged tissue may drain, and this may save the overlying skin. At a later stage, if there is more than a 10 mm area of obvious skin damage this should be excised along with the devitalized subcutaneous tissue. This may well limit the amount of slough that would otherwise be the outcome. A small split-skin graft is taken at the same time and stored at 4°C for application when the defect is considered receptive.

The real problem in such a situation is that the patient is usually so ill that matters such as a small amount of skin loss on the dorsum of the hand are insignificant initially, but when the patient survives the presence of the slough on the back of the hand may be a major issue. This may require resection and grafting, and it is important throughout the development of any such damage that the patient, or alternatively the patient's rela-

tives, should be kept informed at all times, so that unnecessary claims for negligence do not arise.

PIP JOINT COVER

The considerations of skin cover in the PIP joint area cannot be separated from the risk of complications affecting the extensor apparatus and the periarticular soft tissues. This usually takes the form of initial oedema, which is later consolidated into scar tissue. Other chapters deal with burns to the area and specific flaps to meet the requirements of skin cover.

The natural tendency of the injured PIP joint is to assume a position of moderate flexion, and this, combined with the general effects of trauma, can rapidly lead to fixation of the finger in this position. Furthermore, damage to the extensor tendon may render the middle slip ineffectual in actively extending the joint from this position. The lateral bands also have a tendency to migrate anteriorly in these circumstances, resulting in their line of force shifting anteriorly to the axis of the joint and thus exacerbating the flexion deformity.

Treatment in principle is directed at the preservation of the viability of the extensor tendon and its adjacent lateral bands. Early active mobilization of the proximal IP joint is advisable to prevent the adhesion of a complex arrangement of extensor tendons and periarticular structures. To permit early mobilization, tendons must be covered by good quality skin, ideally provided by a local flap which must be arranged so that the movement is not restricted. Some limitation of movement in the MP and DIP joints is acceptable, but it is essential that the PIP joint recovers an almost full range of movement, and this recovery of flexion is the key to recovery of digital function. There is a natural tendency for the PIP joint to become immobile in a semiflexed position, and for this reason it must not be allowed to rest in this position for any length of time. The elective resting position must be close to full extension. It is easier for the patient to recover flexion from an almost extended position than to recover extension from a semiflexed position. In the early stages of mobilization passive assistance is required, but gradually the patient should be capable of controlling these movements actively. This is one area of rehabilitation where the hand therapist plays a particularly important role, in the provision of various forms of splintage to meet the requirements of immobilization in extension, alternating with active flexion, and the supervision of this to a successful outcome.

Slowness of healing or secondary healing invites added scarring which is superimposed on the natural tendency of the area to produce subcutaneous scar tissue, and it is therefore essential that any form of grafting or flap cover is achieved with primary wound healing and without complications. This objective, plus the provision of a form of cover that does not physically restrict the movement of the joint, is the basis of functional recovery.

SKIN COVER IN THE NAIL AREA

The nail functions as a part of the skeleton of the terminal phalanx in providing stability for the pulp at either side and at the apex. The nail also plays a significant cosmetic role particularly in females, and in many young women this far exceeds its functional role. The nail is derived from separate sources of keratin, which combine to form the nail proper. Any of these may be damaged, or they may become separated from their other constituent parts, producing considerable variations in the final shape and disposition of the nail.

The object of treatment should be the restoration of the nail components in their pre-injury positions. Provided there is little or no loss of the germinal components of the nailbed, and provided the nailfold space can be kept open, then an acceptable new nail should grow. If less than one-third of the nail remains it is probably better totally removed. Care must be taken to make sure the removal is complete, otherwise troublesome remnants will require further ablative surgery. Excised nail, the bed of which is grafted, gives an acceptable functional and cosmetic repair. Frequently crush injuries lead to the displacement of parts of the germinal nail area, which continue to develop in a displaced relationship if not corrected at the time of injury. This leads to a variety of distortions, some of which can be particularly disfig-

uring and also cause a considerable nuisance and discomfort.

The nail, which is often poorly understood by surgeons, usually suffers the further disadvantage of being treated by relatively junior doctors. There are two basic requirements in the management of nail trauma. These concern the nailfold space and the supraperiosteal component of the nailbed. The space under the nailfold, which is lined on either side by nail germinal cells and normally separated by the distally growing nail, must not be allowed to coalesce. The space should be kept open either by the reinserted nail or a substitute spacer, until sufficient further proper nail keratin is generated in the space to retain the separation of its component surfaces.

The nailbed element, which is inseparable from the dorsal periosteum, must be repaired as accurately as possible and without further trauma. A transverse scar must be so fine and well healed that the advancing nail will obtain attachment to its bed distal to the scar. It may be necessary to mobilize the nailbed before carefully trimming its edge, and to suture with a 6/0 monofilament non-absorbable suture. The advancing nail often fails to gain attachment to the nailbed distal to a widened scar, and the premature separation of the nail and its bed from this level distally persists and is very difficult to correct. Planing machine accidents in which the nail and part of the adjacent bone are removed may also result in the loss of the insertion of the distal interphalangeal joint extensor tendon, and in this case the joint should be arthrodesed in about 20° flexion. The defect, whether or not there has been damage to the extensor tendon, is best treated by a small reverse-dermis flap taken from the adjacent finger and overgrafted. Alternatively, a small cross-arm flap can provide a suitable replacement cover that is not too restrictive and not too bulky. A groin flap in this situation is too bulky and also quite difficult to devise for such a small area, and is generally better reserved for much bigger defects. Submammary flaps are safe and reasonably convenient, but also suffer from being rather bulky. They may produce considerable chest-wall disfigurement, particularly if there is a tendency towards hypertrophic scar formation. The flap-graft (Chapter 6) may provide the answer to this problem.

CAR SCRAPE INJURIES

These occur to front-seat occupants of cars which overturn with the side windows open. The hand is usually trapped between the top of the door and the ground. The injury is a mixture of abrasion, compression and rotation. A variable amount of damage to the skin on the dorsum of the hand is encountered, the wound is invariably grossly contaminated with road debris, and quite frequently the extensor tendons are shredded. The index and middle-finger metacarpals are more often involved with severely comminuted, and usually anteriorly displaced, fractures. The management of these involves the stable reduction of the fractures, the complete debridement of foreign and dead tissues from the wound, and a conservative debridement of the extensor tendons. These are invariably exposed, without paratenon cover, and require vascularized cover. Usually a flap is required and rarely is it possible to arrange the remaining viable skin to cover the exposed tendons satisfactorily. Each case, however, is treated on its merits. Formerly, a groin flap was the customary means of cover for such an injury,

but more recently, the radial forearm flap, or forearm fascial flap overgrafted with split skin (see Chapter 4), has been used in preference to the rather bulky groin flap, which invariably requires thinning. The fractures must be accurately reduced and held sufficiently to allow early active movement. One of the main problems in such an injury arises from the adhesion of the damaged tendons to the underlying bone and overlying cover. Anticipating this, it is advisable where possible to introduce some layer of viable tissue to separate the fracture from the tendon. The tendon may become adherent to the edges of the flap, but this is a much easier problem to deal with later. It is because of the adhesion problems that early active movement is advised, and this cannot be achieved unless the fractures that often accompany these injuries are satisfactorily dealt with initially.

Skin, the largest organ of the body, is indispensable and is nowhere more important than on the hand. This chapter sets out to show that no matter how excellent the repair, replacement or reconstruction of other components, the result will be poor if proper skin cover is not achieved.

REFERENCES

Coleman J S and Anson B J 1961 Arterial patterns in the hand based upon a study of 650 specimens. Surgery, Gynaecology and Obstetrics 113: 409–424

Bevin A G and Hothem A L 1978 The use of silicone rods under split-thickness skin grafts for reconstruction of flexor tendon injuries. Hand 10: 254–258

14 Skin loss in the palm and web spaces

The anatomical construction of the hand is responsible for the differences between the dorsum and the palm of the hand in the treatment of skin defects and the development of scar contractures. The dorsal skin is thin and much more pliable and mobile against the underlying structures, while the palmar skin is thick and fixed by fibrous septa. For this reason, the shifting of local skin in the palm is only possible to a limited extent. Furthermore the indications for and the operative technique of skin cover in the palm are influenced by the high mechanical stresses during almost all activities of the hand, so that thin split-thickness skin grafts do not provide adequate skin cover.

The prevention and treatment of scar contractures play an important part in any surgical intervention in the palm, and especially in the web spaces. While the tendency for scar tissue to contract will generally lead to tension, or even contracture, in a scar, the danger of such developments is much greater in the palmar aspect and the web spaces of the hand. The reason for this is the ease with which joints yield to the pull of shrinking scar tissue both towards a flexed position and into adduction. The thenar crease is also a joint crease, and a transverse scar running from the thenar to the hypothenar eminence will cause scar contracture by flexing the carpometacarpal joints of the thumb and little finger.

The development of scar contractures should be avoided by the correct placement of surgical incisions. Any longitudinal incision on the flexor aspect of a digit, and any transverse incision in the web spaces or in the middle of the palm, must be avoided or interrupted by a Z-plasty. The same guiding principle applies to longitudinal or transverse wound margins in the same areas resulting from the excision of a scar or tumour, or from a traumatic skin defect. Such a wound margin should be interrupted by darts or by small local flaps before the wound is closed either by direct suture or by a free graft or even a flap (see Figs 14.6 and 14.7). If this is not done, avoidable scar contractures will need correction at a second operation (Fig. 14.1).

The prevention of scar contractures is of particular importance in the hands of children. Here one has to anticipate the development of contraction at *any* localization in the hand, not only on the flexor aspect and the web spaces. Therefore any longitudinal scar has to be avoided by zig-zag incisions or the interruption of straight wound margins.

SKIN COVER IN THE PALM

The skin of the palm needs to withstand high pressure and shearing forces, so that only full-thickness skin grafts or flaps will give sufficient cover. Thin split-thickness skin grafts are acceptable only as a temporary wound closure in infected or irradiated wounds, and have to be replaced later by thicker skin. Most authors concur with this opinion, although Pensler et al (1988) found no functional difference between full-thickness and split-thickness skin grafts in the burned palm of children. Sensation is also of great importance, so that large skin flaps are usually not appropriate.

Skin cover with local skin

Local skin is the best source of cover in the

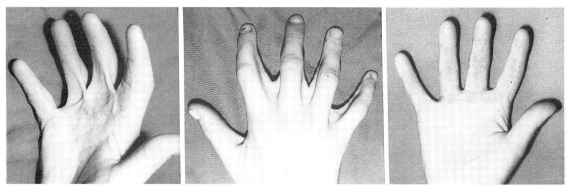

Fig. 14.1 Scar contractures of the web spaces of the fingers caused by straight margins of split-thickness skin grafts used for cover of localized burn wounds (left and centre). Correction by multiple Z-plasties (right).

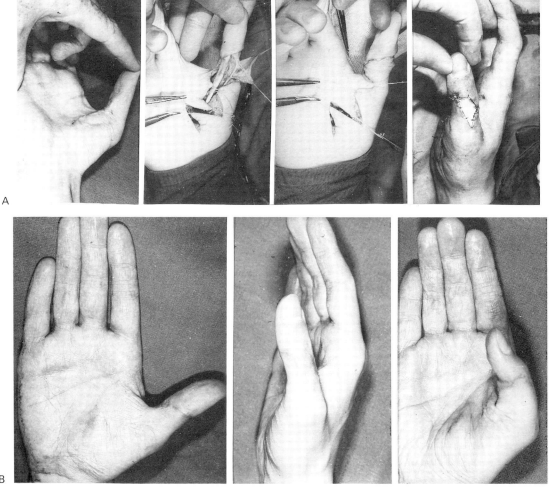

Fig. 14.2A Longitudinal scar contracture of the thumb following inappropriate extension of the laceration for primary repair of flexor pollicis longus (left). Closure of the defect resulting from scar excision and tenolysis, with dissection of the neurovascular bundles, using Z-plasties and a transposition flap from the dorsum of the thumb (centre). Cover of the donor site with a thick split-thickness skin graft (right). **B** The result, showing full extension and radial abduction, a useful range of flexion and good aesthetic appearance.

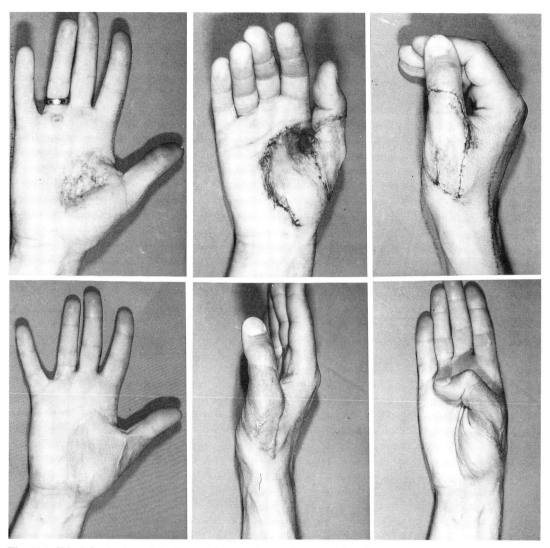

Fig. 14.3 Skin defect in the radial palm and thenar eminence due to excision of a tumour, covered by a large transposition flap which includes the intact skin of the thenar eminence and the dorsum of the thumb. The donor site was closed with a thick split-thickness skin graft. The functional and aesthetic result was good.

palm because its texture and quality are the same. Unfortunately local skin is only available to a limited extent, due to the abrupt change in the characteristics of the skin on the relatively narrow borders of the palm and the lack of pliability of the palmar skin. Therefore only small defects can be repaired with a flap of adjacent local skin. This may be indicated if tendons or neurovascular structures are exposed (Fig. 14.2), or the defect is too deep to allow the use of a full-thickness skin graft. On the ulnar half of the palm a defect can be

covered by a transposition flap from the ulnar border, including some dorsal skin. Alternatively an island flap may be raised on the hypothenar eminence, with a distally based pedicle of the common digital artery of the little finger with reversed flow, as described by Kojima et al (1990).

On the radial side of the palm the skin of the thenar eminence and the dorsum of the thumb can be included in a transposition flap, providing skin cover in the lateral palm (Fig. 14.3). The flap

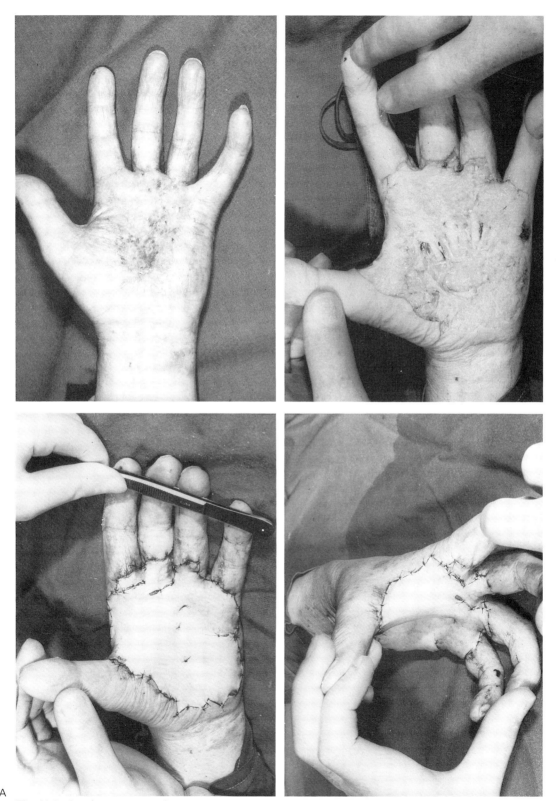

A

Fig. 14.4 (caption on next page)

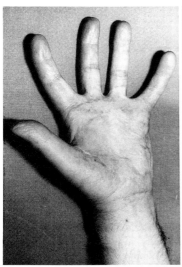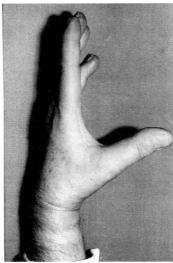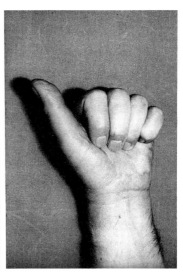

Fig. 14.4 A Radiation injury of the skin of the palm. Following excision there was enough subcutaneous tissue to allow the use of a full-thickness skin graft. Not the avoidance of any straight wound margins, especially in the web spaces. **B** The result shows an almost full range of motion and no scar tension.

must be elevated with careful preservation of the arteries, veins and cutaneous nerve branches, so that blood and nerve supply remain undisturbed (see also the dorsal rotation flap for widening of the first web space, p. 172).

Skin cover with free skin grafts

Because thin split-thickness skin grafts are not appropriate for the function of the palmar skin, their use is indicated only for temporary skin cover in severely infected wounds, or to cover defects following malignant tumour excision to observe for local recurrence. Full-thickness skin grafts can give excellent functional and cosmetic results if they are applied in the correct manner, even if they are quite extensive. They are indicated in more superficial defects such as radiation skin injuries; in these insidious precancerous pathological conditions, all the skin layers are involved but the subcutaneous tissue is mostly intact (Fig. 14.4). In these cases the prevention of later scar contractures is very important: the wound margins must follow a zig-zag course, and extensions of the graft should reach the opposite side of a web space (Buck-Gramcko 1962, 1968). A full take of the graft is the reward for meticulous

haemostasis and careful dressing technique with a tie-over dressing. Smaller grafts in the palm also require a tie-over dressing to provide uniform slight compression and immobilization.

Skin cover with flaps

Flaps are rarely indicated as cover for palmar defects, but may be needed for deep or large defects which expose the tendons and neurovascular bundles; these wounds are unsuitable for free grafts, and adjacent skin may not be available. The indications and techniques have recently been summarized by Lister (1988).

As an *island flap* the radial forearm flap (see Chapter 4) can be used, either as a fasciocutaneous flap or by taking fascia alone and providing skin cover with a split-thickness skin graft.

Free skin flaps with microvascular anastomosis (see Chapter 7) demand microsurgical expertise; they are indicated only under special individual circumstances. Flaps with a thin layer of subcutaneous tissue, such as the lateral arm (Chapter 8) or scapular flaps, are preferred.

The conventional method of skin transportation, the *distant flap*, still has indications (see Chapter 5). Distant flaps are the most reliable form of skin cover, but they have the disadvantage of requiring at least two stages, and an uncomfortable position for the 3 weeks in between. Where microsurgical expertise is not available, or when free flaps are contraindicated, distant flaps can be used either as random or as axial pattern flaps. The cross-arm flap, abdominal flap or groin flap may also be indicated, to provide preliminary soft-tissue cover before complex reconstructive procedures such as thumb reconstruction or toe transplantation.

Open palm technique in Dupuytren's contracture

It may be surprising to find a paragraph on *not* closing an open wound in a book on skin cover; McCash (1964) challenged the surgical rule to close all open wounds: this is mentioned here to stress the fact that the open palm technique is applicable only in Dupuytren's contracture. In contrast to skin defects caused by traumatic skin loss or by excision of tumours or scar tissue in the palm, the gaping wound in Dupuytren's contracture does not represent real skin loss, but is caused by preoperative shrinkage of the skin in the presence of a flexion contracture in the metacarpophalangeal joints. This shrinkage cannot be reversed immediately at operation, but the steady pull of granulation tissue over the course of 2 or 3 weeks can do so. The end result is a linear transverse scar in the distal palm.

Although the open palm technique has the advantage of preventing haematoma, and the avoidance of both oedema and restriction of motion, thereby allowing early active exercises and hand baths, it is not applicable in cases of real skin loss. Here the healing by granulation will result in the formation of much more scar tissue and flexion contracture, and not in extension of the preoperatively shrunken skin.

SKIN COVER IN THE WEB SPACES

The web spaces are relatively small, but they are functionally very important areas of the hand. Their mobility is essential for full abduction of the

digits, especially in the case of the thumb. Their narrowing by scar tissue will interfere considerably with the function of the hand, and therefore the prevention as well as the release of these adduction contractures is an important part of plastic surgery of the hand.

Because of the difference in width of the web spaces of the fingers compared to the first web space, methods applicable to all or to the second to fourth web spaces are mentioned first. The special characteristics of the first web space will follow in a separate section.

Skin cover with local skin

Open wounds in the depths of web spaces occur infrequently, so that scar contractures are more likely to require correction on the palmar or the dorsal aspects of the web. The middle part of the web and the skin over the proximal part of the proximal phalanx are usually intact, and can therefore be used as a source of local flaps. As a rule the procedures are also applicable to partial webbing in incomplete syndactyly.

Almost all methods are Z-plasties or modified Z-plasties, in combination with transposition flaps. A simple Z-plasty may sometimes fulfil the requirements, but better contouring of the web is usually obtained through the use of additional Z-plasties or small local flaps. Most of these methods are modifications of the 'jumping man' procedure which was first described by Mustardé (1963) for correction of epicanthic folds (Fig. 14.5).

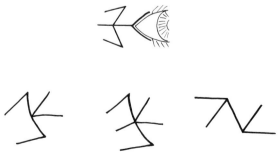

Fig. 14.5 Schematic drawing of the original design for Mustardé's 'jumping man' (top), the butterfly-plasty (Shaw et al 1972, 1973), (left), the five-flap Z-plasty (Hirshowitz et al 1975) (lower centre) and the four-flap Z-plasty (Woolf and Broadbent 1972) (right).

Chapman et al (1987) have given Mustardé the full credit for this procedure – his name is not usually mentioned in the hand surgical literature. Modifications have been published, including the 'butterfly-plasty' (Shaw et al 1972), the 'trident plasty' (Glicenstein & Bonnefous 1975), the 'five-flap Z-plasty' (Hirshowitz et al 1975), and the 'VM-plasty' (Alexander et al 1982). The M-V flap (Lewis et al 1988) is slightly different and can be combined with the transposition of adjacent skin as described by Bunnell (1956), Tanzer (1948), MacDougal et al (1976), Beasley (1981), and

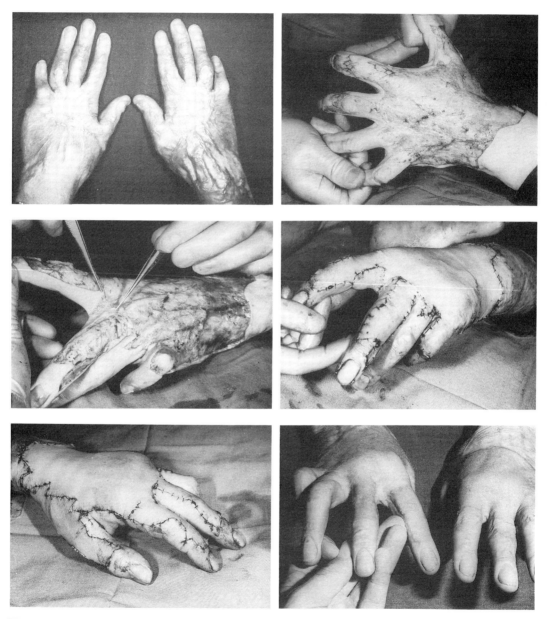

Fig. 14.6 Dorsal burn scar with web-space contracture. Excision left a well-vascularized bed, suitable for a full-thickness skin graft. The transverse wounds in the web spaces (upper row right) had to be interrupted by a vertical incision in each as far as the palm, to accept an extension of the graft. This, together with the interdigitated wound margins (even between two skin grafts as over the first metacarpal, below left) will prevent tension in the surrounding scars, allowing an excellent result (below right).

Colson (1985). Smith and Harrison (1982) described the 'seagull flap', which was used in three adjacent fingers by Matthews and Morgan (1987). Ostrowski et al (1991) demonstrated the release of a web contracture by means of a dorsal rectangular and two palmar triangular local flaps. The author prefers the butterfly-plasty (Fig. 14.5), often using the modification developed by Hirshowitz et al (1975). An additional skin graft is necessary only in very rare cases.

Skin cover with free skin grafts

Coverage of web-space wounds with skin grafts is rarely indicated, because at least part of the web-space skin is usually uninjured. This normal skin will usually cover the lateral parts of the web space, so that the graft has to be inserted in the middle. In most cases such a graft is an extension of a large graft on the dorsum (Fig. 14.6) or the palm (Fig. 14.3). Grafts are inserted in this way more for the prevention of later scar contracture by avoiding a transverse suture line, than as cover of a real skin defect resulting from traumatic loss. The graft may consist of either full- or split-thickness skin, depending on which is being used for the main graft on the palm or the dorsum of the hand.

Skin cover with island flaps

Although the first reported use of an island flap was probably by Monks in 1898 (but he did not call his flap for reconstruction of the lower eyelid by that name), and the term 'island flap' seems to have been coined by Esser in 1917, it required greater specialization in the field of hand surgery, and more expertise in the dissection of small anatomical structures and the shifting of tissues, for island flaps to enter routine use in hand surgery. Moberg was the first to use an island flap which included sensory innervation (Moberg 1964). The method was refined by Littler (1956) and by Tubiana and Duparc (1961) and Tubiana et al (1960).

Some relatively small island flaps have been developed for skin cover in the web spaces. In most designs the vascular pedicle is relatively short. The earliest flap of this kind was the flag flap, known also as the French flap – not only referring to the colour sequence it sometimes shows (first red, then white, and finally blue), but related more to its first description in France. Vilain (1952) and later Iselin and Gosse (1962) raised this flap on the dorsum of a finger with a small skin bridge, including the blood vessels, as a pedicle. This was recommended also in their English publication in 1973 (Vilain & Dupuis 1973, Iselin 1973). Later the flag flap was refined for use as an island flap, based on either the dorsal metacarpal artery or on the dorsal branch of the palmar digital artery and the surrounding veins (Lister 1981, 1985, 1988). This pedicle provides a far wider range of applications in the web space and the palmar and dorsal aspects of the proximal phalanges of the same or an adjacent digit. The venous dorsal digital flap of Foucher and Norris (1988) is similar, but based only on a pedicle of several dorsal digital veins.

A somewhat wider arc of rotation is available with more proximal island flaps based on the dorsal metacarpal arteries. Anatomical studies on vascularization by Kuhlmann (1978), Oberlin and Le Quang (1985), Earley (1986), Earley and Milner (1987) and Oberlin et al (1988) have shown a rich network of anastomoses between the dorsal metacarpal arteries (especially the second) and the palmar digital arteries. This not only explains the clinical success of distal flag flaps, but also forms the vascular basis for island flaps with a distal or proximal vascular pedicle. The second dorsal metacarpal artery flap seems to be of particular value (Earley & Milner 1987). It is useful for covering defects particularly in the first web space, but can also reach other web spaces and proximal phalanges (Arria & Gilbert 1990, Maruyama 1990, Quaba & Davison 1990, Small & Brennen 1990).

The 'kite' flap has a similar vascular basis (Foucher et al 1978, Foucher & Braun 1979, Marin-Braun et al 1988), and is better suited to defects of the thumb than the first web space.

Hilgenfeldt originally described this flap in 1950 and again in 1964. He used it with a skin pedicle, as have Buck-Gramcko (1961) as a primary procedure and Kuhn (1961) for secondary reconstruction. Holevich (1963) and Small and Brennen (1988) have used this flap as an island

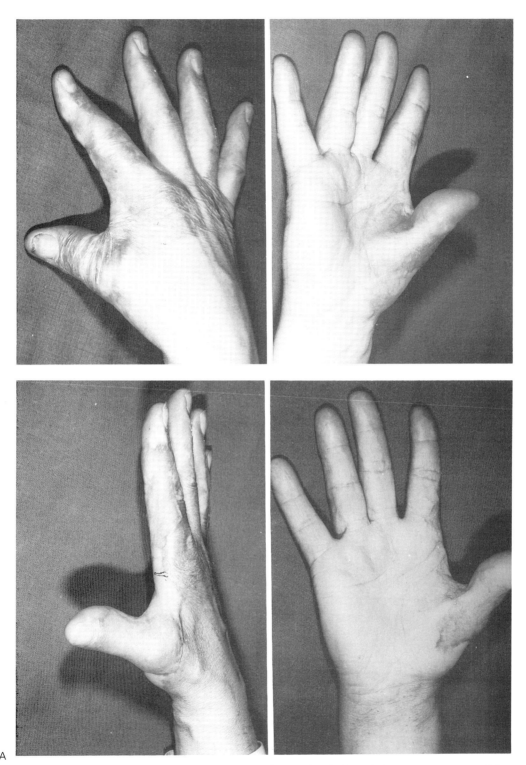

Fig. 14.7 To obtain the result shown in the lower two photographs (**A**) from the burn scar contracture of the first web space including parts of the thumb and index finger (upper two photographs in **A**) it was necessary to interrupt straight wound margins by darts or local sliding flaps (**B**), so that no scar tension will develop.

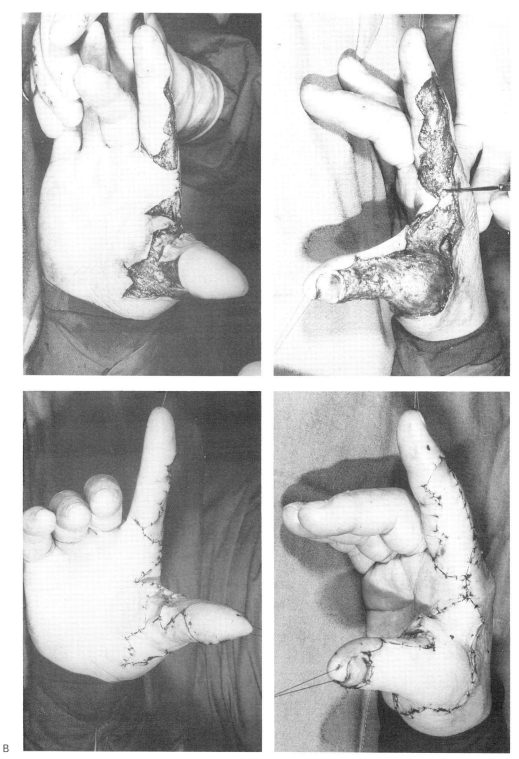

B

Fig. 14.7 Cont'd.

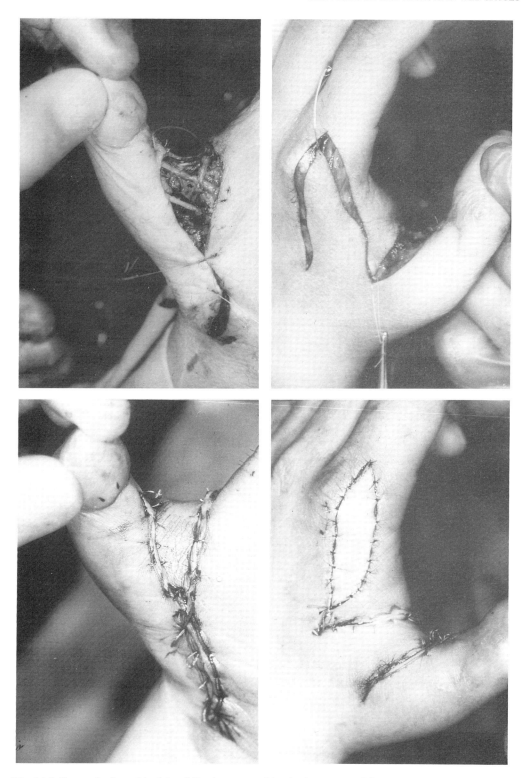

Fig. 14.8 Cover of a deep skin defect following scar excision in the contracted first web, with nerve grafting for the thumb, by a transposition flap from the index finger ray with full-thickness skin graft for the donor site.

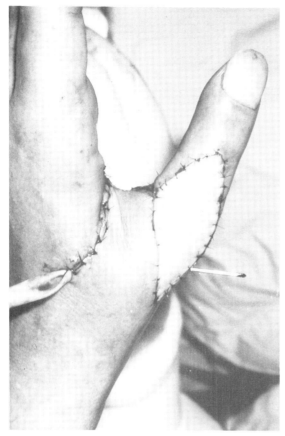

Fig. 14.9 Cover of a released first web space by a transposition flap from the dorsum of the thumb. (Courtesy of G D Lister M D)

flap, while several other authors have applied the cross-finger flap technique (Buck-Gramcko 1988).

Other island flaps with a more proximal vascular pedicle can be applied to all web spaces. They have been described in recent years as a result of the continuous search for new flaps. In addition to the important radial forearm flap (Chapter 4) the distally or proximally based posterior interosseous flap should be mentioned (Masquelet & Penteado 1987, Costa & Soutar 1988, Zancolli & Angrigiani 1988), and the ulnar artery flap (Becker & Gilbert 1988, Guimberteau et al 1988).

Special characteristics of the first web space

The first web space of the hand has much more functional importance than the others, because an

adduction contracture of the thumb will greatly interfere with the total function of the hand. Adduction contractures of the thumb may be caused by such congenital malformations as hypoplasia of the thumb, or syndactyly between thumb and index finger, direct trauma to the skin and/or muscles of this area, burns, trauma to the forearm with nerve damage or ischaemia, faulty immobilization in an adducted position or with strangulation, and by Dupuytren's disease.

The treatment of almost all types of adduction contracture of the thumb requires scar excision, and skin cover once the release is complete. In principle the same methods are applicable as in the other web spaces, but the difference lies in the amount of skin required. The width of the first web space requires much more skin, and there is a great need for pliability and tolerance of wear and shearing stress.

Skin grafts

For these reasons split-thickness skin grafts are rarely indicated, and then only as temporary skin cover, which has to be replaced later by skin of better quality. Full-thickness skin grafts have their special indications in burn contractures in which all deep tissues are intact. Here the same rules have to be observed as in the other web spaces and the palm, to prevent later tension in marginal scars. Transverse wound margins in the web space have to be interrupted by darts or by small local sliding flaps (Fig. 14.7).

Local skin flaps

If deeper structures are exposed a flap is required. In very exceptional cases the filleted skin of an otherwise severely damaged index finger may be used, and several more standardized local flaps have particular value for the first web space. When the defect is not too large, a transposition flap from the dorsum of either the index finger or the thumb is useful. This type of flap is usually well vascularized, but necessitates a skin graft to cover the donor site, as do all transposition flaps (Fig. 14.8). Some authors prefer the dorsum of the thumb as the donor site (Thomine 1971, Strauch 1975, Blauth 1976, Sandzén 1982, Lister

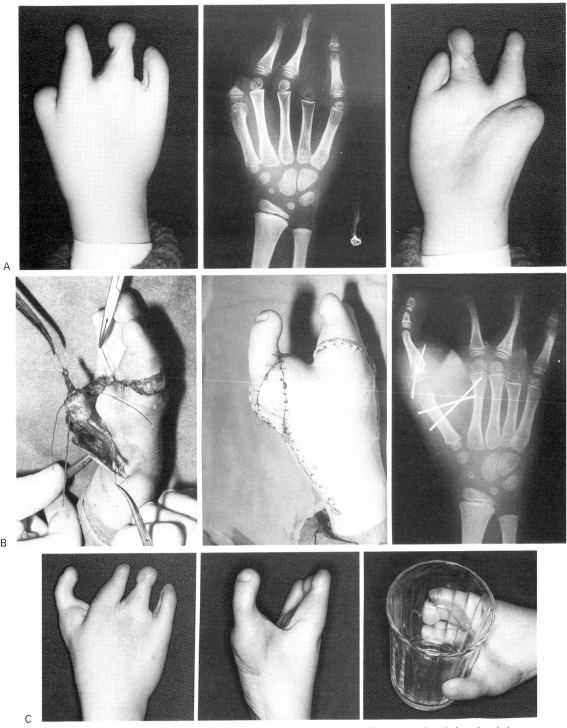

Fig. 14.10 The right hand of a girl aged 6 years with ring constriction syndrome. The acrosyndactyly has already been separated elsewhere, with amputation of the ring finger stump; the partially absent thumb is fixed in an adducted position (**A**). At the same time as transplantation of the right second toe the first ray was released and temporarily fixed in abduction with two crossed K-wires. The defect in the first web space was covered by an advancement-rotation flap from the dorsum (**B**). The result 4 years later shows the wide abduction of the thumb and the almost invisible scar on the dorsum (**C**).

1985; Fig. 14.9), while others take the flap from the index finger and part of the dorsal metacarpal region (Littler 1959, Brand 1964, Beasley 1967, Spinner 1969, Brown 1972, Joshi 1974, Tubiana 1985). This transposition flap from the dorsal aspect of the index finger ray is described by Chanson and Michon (1979) and by Thomine (1985) as the 'lambeau de Tessier', but no bibliographic reference was given. Strickland (1982) has extended the dorsal transposition flap to the middle finger ray, as have Abe et al (1982) and Tajima (1985), although both Strickland (1982) and Brown (1972) have incorrectly described it as a rotation flap. Flatt and Wood (1970) preferred multiple dorsal rotation flaps and Caroli and Zanasi (1989) used a combination of a dorsal and a palmar flap. Excellent reviews are given by Furnas (1985) and by Glicenstein and Leclercq (1985).

Dorsal rotation advancement flap For larger defects the author's preferred technique is a dorsal flap which has features of a rotation and an advancement flap (Fig. 14.10). This flap is particularly indicated in children with thumb/ index syndactyly (Buck-Gramcko 1991) or with an adducted position of the thumb in other congenital malformations (Riordan 1976), but it is also valuable for traumatic defects (Fig. 14.11). The tip of the flap is usually located on the dorsal aspect of the proximal phalanx of the index finger, but not too far distally, to allow direct closure of the donor site. The use of an additional full-thickness skin graft is only necessary sometimes in adults, in whom the skin is less pliable than in children, or in children with a narrowed dorsum as a result of oligodactyly.

There are two important technical details in the procedure. First, the flap should be raised with careful preservation of the nerve and blood vessel branches. Although it is essential to mobilize the flap adequately to allow advancement and rotation far enough into the web space for the tip to reach palmar skin, the supplying branches should not be divided, but freed by meticulous dissection. The other important practical detail is the fixation of the thumb ray in full abduction (in most cases in a position midway between radial and palmar abduction) by means of two crossed Kirschner

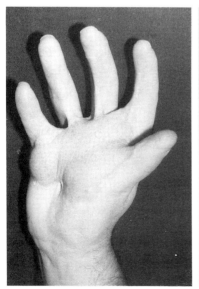 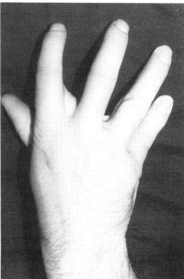 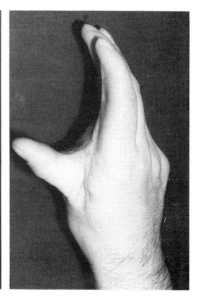

A

Fig. 14.11 Adduction contracture of the thumb due to insufficient abdominal skin flap cover for burn wounds. (**A**) Following release of the thumb the widened web space was covered by a rotation flap from the dorsum. Note the careful preservation of supplying vessels and nerve branches (**B**, above right). The tip of the flap must reach the opposite side of the hand to prevent subsequent scar tension in the web space (**B**, below). The donor site was closed directly with the help of a back-cut (Burow's triangle). The result 5 years later shows not only a wide first web space covered with normal skin, but also very little scar formation on the dorsum (**C**).

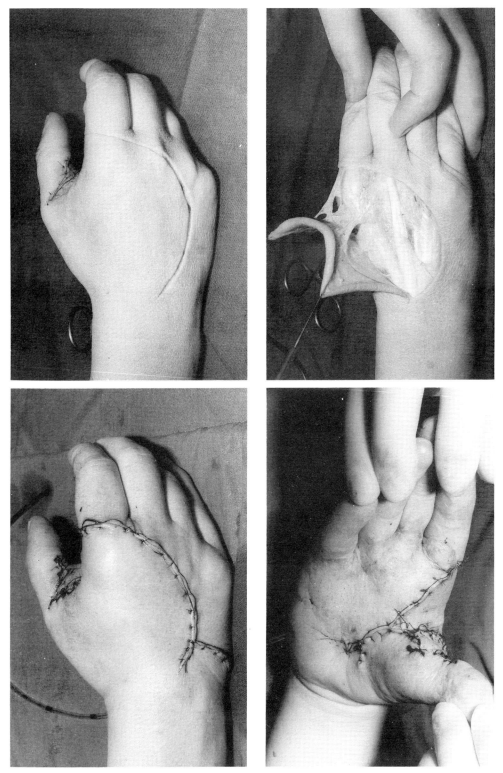

B

Fig. 14.11 Cont'd.

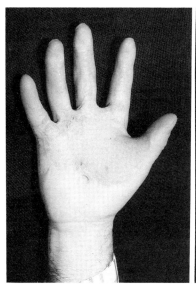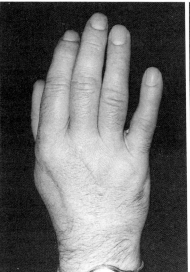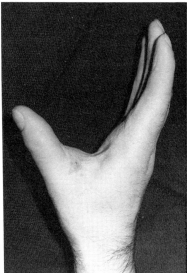

C

Fig. 14.11 Contd.

wires between the first and second metacarpal bones. Otherwise there is a tendency for the thumb ray to fall back into an adducted position. This would compress the distal part of the flap and compromise its blood supply.

The results are very satisfying if all these essential features are observed. The dorsal skin becomes pliable again within a few months; in most cases the scar is almost invisible 2 years postoperatively (Figs 14.10, 14.11). The new first web space is lined with skin of the best quality, able to withstand the stresses of daily life.

Z-plasties In cases of less severe contracture or partial syndactyly in which it is not necessary to bring so much additional skin to the web space, which only needs to be widened and deepened, local skin transposition by Z-plasty is a simple but effective method. Sometimes a single Z-plasty is sufficient, but in many cases one of the more sophisticated Z-plasties has to be used (see Fig. 14.5). In these, several triangular flaps with angles of less than 60° are transposed to obtain more length. Although originally described by Limberg (cited by Furnas 1965, Limberg 1966 and 1967) they became better known as a result of later publications. This type of Z-plasty was called 'Z rectifiés' by Iselin (1962; also Buck-Gramcko

1968, Wintsch et al 1971), '120° Z-plasty' (Lister & Milward 1976) or 'four-flap Z-plasty' (Woolf & Broadbent 1972). Further modifications based on Mustardé's 'jumping man' principle are mentioned above. Additional procedures that have been described are five-flap (Rousso 1975, Chanson & Michon 1979) or even six-flap Z-plasties (Mir y Mir 1973).

The author's preferred method is a four-flap Z-plasty (see Fig. 14.5), which solves skin cover problems if the skin contacture is superficial and the thumb is not adducted.

Distant flaps

The amount of skin sometimes necessary in a severe adduction contracture of the first web space creates the need for the use of distant flaps. Indications still exist today, especially where microsurgical expertise is not available. The opposite upper arm has been recommended by Mutz (1972) as a donor site for the diamond-shaped flap, while two triangular flaps have been used by Bonola and Fiocchi (1975) as well as by Yeschua et al (1977) and Teich-Alasia and Barberis (1972). In most cases the lower abdomen or groin have been used as a donor site (Bunnell 1956, Beasley 1967, 1981, Colson & Janvier

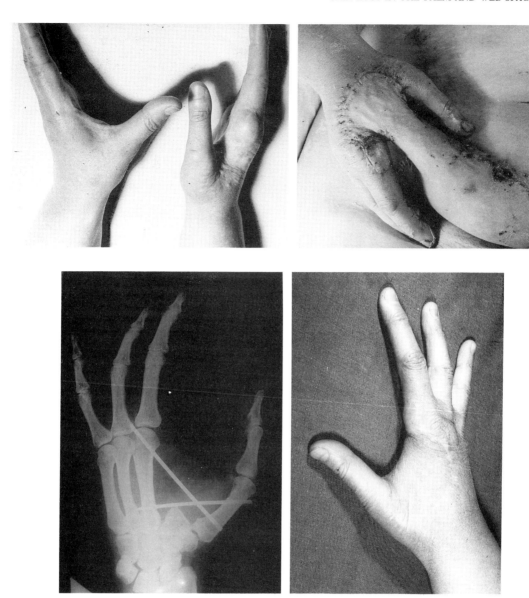

Fig. 14.12 Adduction contracture of the thumb in a case of crush injury with loss of the second ray. Following scar excision the adducted thumb was temporarily fixed with crossed K-wires and the widened first web space covered with an abdominal tube pedicle flap. The result is excellent, due, to some extent, to the primary defatting of the skin flap.

1966, Howard 1950, Lister 1988, Littler 1959, Miura 1979 with paired flaps). The procedure is safe, but it requires two stages with an interval of 3 weeks. The results are usually satisfactory, especially if the layer of subcutaneous tissue is not too thick. Either a direct abdominal flap or a tube pedicle are possible (Figs 14.12, 14.13).

Island flaps

Most of the island flaps taken from the hand itself offer too little skin, so only flaps from the forearm are suitable. The best known and most valuable flap is the radial forearm flap, which provides enough skin even for large defects (see Chapter 4). It is also the flap of choice for medium-sized

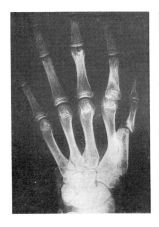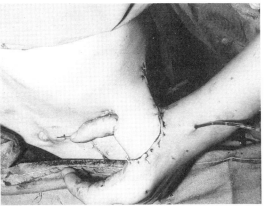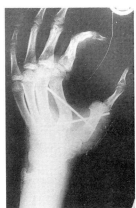

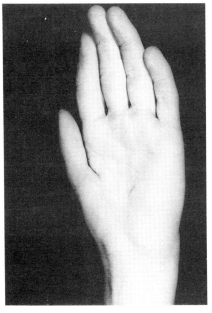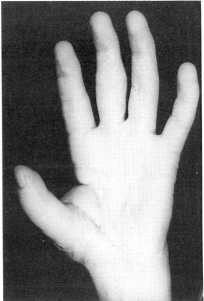

Fig. 14.13 Severe adduction contracture of the thumb following and explosive injury (left above and below). After release and temporary K-wire fixation the defect in the widened first web space was covered with a direct abdominal skin flap (above centre and right). The result shows good abduction of the thumb (below right).

defects when dorsal hand skin is not available due to scarring (Fig. 14.14). Other possible island flaps are mentioned above in the section on skin cover in the finger web spaces (p. 166).

Free flaps

Free flaps are rarely indicated as skin cover for the first web space, and there is a risk that they may be used by overenthusiastic microsurgeons with in-

adequate knowledge of the above-mentioned 'conventional' methods. The indication does exist in cases with multiple scarred areas on both the dorsum of the hand and the forearm, so that no local skin and no island flap donor sites are available. Reviews of the various possibilities are given by Hing et al (1985) and by MacLeod et al (1985). Scheker et al (1988) prefer the lateral arm flap, Büchler et al (1981) the dorsalis pedis flap (see also Chapters 8 and 10).

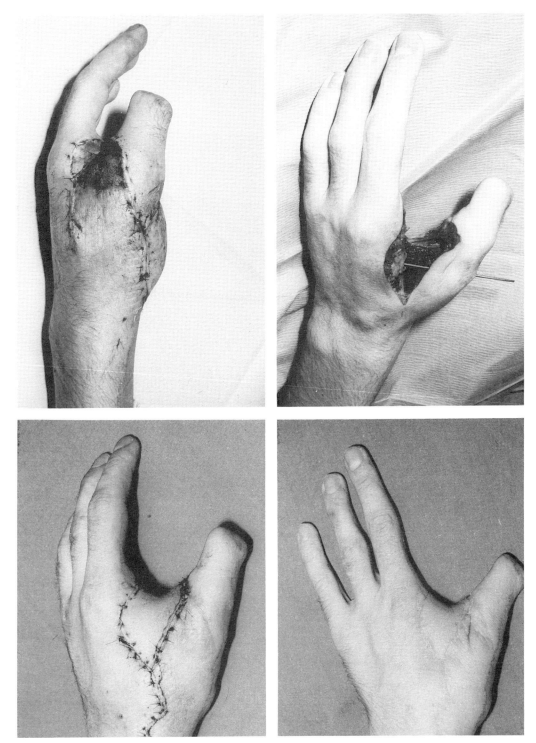

Fig. 14.14 Adduction contracture of the thumb following thumb reconstruction by transposition of the partially amputated index finger, caused by necrosis of the dorsal web flap (above left). Following scar excision the released new thumb was fixed with K-wires (above right), and the 'empty' first web was covered by a radial forearm island flap (below left). As a result the reconstructed thumb regained the necessary wide abduction (below right).

REFERENCES

Abe M, Ikeda K, Yasunaga H et al 1982 Surgical treatment of the thumb. Proceedings of the 25th Annual Meeting of the Japanese Society for Surgery of the Hand, Tokyo, pp. 27–29

Alexander J W, MacMillan B G, Mariel L 1982 Correction of postburn syndactyly: an analysis of children with introduction of the VM-plasty and postoperative pressure inserts. Plastic and Reconstructive Surgery 70: 345–352

Arria P, Gilbert A 1990 Lambeaux des artères interosseuses dorsales de la main. In: Gilbert A, Masquelet A C, Hentz R V (eds) Les lambeaux artériels pédiculés du membre supérieure. Monographies du GEM, 17, Expansion Scientifique Française, Paris, pp. 121–131

Beasley R W 1967 Principles and techniques of resurfacing operations for hand surgery. Surgical Clinics of North America 47: 389-413

Beasley R W 1981 Secondary repair of burned hands. Clinics in Plastic Surgery 8: 141–162

Becker C, Gilbert A 1988 Le lambeau cubital. Annales de Chirurgie de la Main 7: 136–142

Blauth W 1976 Zur Behandlung der verengten Daumenkommissur mit der 'erweiterten Schwenklappenplastik'. Handchirurgie 8: 71–74

Bonola A, Fiocchi R 1975 Cross-arm double flap in the repair of severe adduction contracture of the thumb. Hand 7: 287–290

Brand P W 1964 Deformity in leprosy. Orthopaedic principles and practical methods of relief. In: Cochrane R G, Frank D T (eds) Leprosy in theory and practice, 2nd edn, John Wright & Sons Ltd., Bristol, pp. 447–496

Brown P W 1972 Adduction–flexion contracture of the thumb. Correction with dorsal rotation flap and release of contracture. Clinical Orthopaedics and Related Research 88: 161–168

Büchler U, Donski P, Tschopp H M 1981 Adduktionskontrakturen der Daumenkommissur: Behandlungsmethoden unter besonderer Berücksichtigung der freien Dorsalis-pedis-Lappenplastik. Therapeutische Umschau 38: 1190–1196

Buck-Gramcko D 1961 Wiederherstellung der Sensibilität bei Teilverlust des Daumens. Langenbecks Archiv für klinische Chirurgie 299: 99–104

Buck-Gramcko D 1962 Plastisch-chirurgische Behandlung von Narbenkontrakturen der Hand. Münchener medizinische Wochenschrift 104: 311–316

Buck-Gramcko D 1968 Deckung von Hautdefekten an der Hand. Chirurgische Praxis 12: 85–94, 263–273

Buck-Gramcko D 1988 Thumb reconstruction after partial amputation of the thumb. In: Tubiana R (ed) The hand. Vol. 111, Saunders, Philadelphia

Buck-Gramcko D 1991 Syndactyly between thumb and index finger. In: Buck-Gramcko D (ed) Congenital malformations of the hand and forearm. Churchill Livingstone, Edinburgh

Bunnell St 1956 Surgery of the hand, 3rd edn. Lippincott, Philadelphia

Caroli A, Zanasi S 1989 First web-space reconstruction by Caroli's technique in congenital hand deformities with severe thumb ray adduction. British Journal of Plastic Surgery 42: 653–659

Chanson L, Michon J 1979 Corrections plastiques des rétractions de la commissure du pouce. Annales de Chirurgie 33: 689-695

Chapman P, Banerjee A, Campbell R C 1987 Extended use of the Mustarde 'dancing man' procedure. British Journal of Plastic Surgery 40: 432–435

Colson P 1985 The laterodigital flap. In: Tubiana R (ed) The hand, Vol. II, pp. 370–383 Saunders, Philadelphia

Colson P, Janvier H 1966 Le dégraissage primaire et total des lambeaux d'autoplastie á distance. Annales de Chirurgie Plastique 11: 11–20

Costa H, Soutar D S 1988 The distally based island posterior interosseous flap. British Journal of Plastic Surgery 41: 221–227

Earley M J 1986 The arterial supply of the thumb, first web and index finger and its surgical application. Journal of Hand Surgery 11B: 163–174

Earley M J, Milner R H 1987 Dorsal metacarpal flaps. British Journal of Plastic Surgery 40: 333–341

Esser J F S 1917 Island flaps. New York Medical Journal 106: 264–265

Flatt A E, Wood V E 1970 Multiple dorsal rotation flaps from the hand for thumb web contractures. Plastic and Reconstructive Surgery 45: 258–262

Foucher G, Braun J-B 1979 A new island flap transfer from the dorsum of the index to the thumb. Plastic and Reconstructive Surgery 63: 344–349

Foucher G, Norris R W 1988 The venous dorsal digital island flap, or the "neutral" flap. British Journal of Plastic Surgery 41: 337–343

Foucher G, Braun J B, Merle M, Sibilly A 1978 Le lambeau 'cerf-volant'. Annales de Chirurgie 32: 593–596

Furnas D W 1965 The tetrahedral Z-plasty. Plastic and Reconstructive Surgery 35: 291-302

Furnas D W 1985 Z-plasties and related procedures for the hand and upper limb. Hand Clinics 1: 649–665

Glicenstein J, Bonnefous G 1975 La plastie en trident. Annales de Chirurgie Plastique 20: 257–260

Glicenstein J, Leclercq C 1985 Skin contracture in the hand. In: Tubiana R (ed) The hand, Vol. II Saunders, Philadelphia

Guimberteau J C, Goin J L, Panconi B, Schuhmacher B 1988 The reverse ulnar artery forearm island flap in hand surgery: 54 cases. Plastic and Reconstructive Surgery 81: 925–932

Hilgenfeldt O 1950 Operativer Daumenersatz und Beseitigung von Greifstörungen. Bei finger-velusten. Ferdinand Enke Verlag, Stuttgart

Hilgenfeldt O 1964 Über einen vielfach verwendungsfähigen, neurovaskulären Lappen zur Behebung von Schäden der radialen Handhälfte. Langenbecks Archiv für klinische Chirurgie 306: 152

Hing D N, Buncke H J, Alpert B S, Gordon L 1985 Free flap coverage of the hand. Hand Clinics 1: 741–758

Hirshowitz B, Karev A, Rousso M 1975 Combined double Z-plasty and Y-V advancement for thumb web contracture. Hand 7: 291–293

Holevich J 1963 A new method of restoring sensibility to the thumb. Journal of Bone and Joint Surgery 45B: 496–505

Howard L D 1950 Contracture of the thumb web. Journal of Bone and Joint Surgery 32A: 267–273

Iselin F 1973 The flag flap. Plastic and Reconstructive Surgery 52: 374–377

Iselin M 1962 La plastie en Z rectifiés. Annales de Chirurgie Plastique 7: 295–298

Iselin M, Gosse L 1962 Le lambeau en drapeau. Son emploi

systématique dans le comblement des pertes de substance limitées des doigts. Annales de Chirurgie Plastique 7: 1–7

Joshi B B 1974 Sensory flaps for the degloved mutilated hand. Hand 6: 247–254

Kojima T, Endo T, Fukumoto K 1990 Reverse vascular pedicle hypothenar island flap. Handchirurgie–Mikrochirurgie–Plastische Chirurgie 22: 137–144

Kuhlmann N 1978 Contribution à l'étude de la vascularisation du dos de la main. Son intérêt pratique. Annales de Chirurgie 32: 587–591

Kuhn H 1961 Reconstruction du pouce par 'lambeau de Hilgenfeldt'. Annales de Chirurgie Plastique 6: 259–268

Lewis R C, Nordyke M D, Duncan K H 1988 Web space reconstruction with a M-V flap. Journal of Hand Surgery 13A: 40–43

Limberg A A 1966 Design of local flaps. In: Gibson T (ed) Modern trends in plastic surgery 2: Butterworth, London

Limberg A A 1967 Planimetrie und Stereometrie der Hautplastik. Gustav Fischer, Jena (in German)

Lister G 1981 The theory of the transposition flap and its practical application in the hand. Clinics in Plastic Surgery 8: 115–127

Lister G 1985 Local flaps to the hand. Hand Clinics 1: 621–640

Lister G D 1988 Skin flaps. In: Green D P (ed) Operative hand surgery, 2nd edn. Churchill Livingstone, New York

Lister G D, Milward T M 1976 Skin contracture of the first web space. Transactions of the Sixth International Congress of Plastic and Reconstructive Surgery, Paris, 24–29 August 1975. Masson, Paris

Littler J W 1956 Neurovascular pedicle transfer of tissue in reconstructive surgery of the hand (proceedings). Journal of Bone and Joint Surgery 38A: 917

Littler J W 1959 The prevention and the correction of adduction contracture of the thumb. Clinical Orthopaedics 13: 182–192

McCash C R 1964 The open palm technique in Dupuytren's contracture. British Journal of Plastic Surgery 17: 271–280

MacDougal B, Wray R C, Weeks P M 1976 Lateral–volar finger flap for the treatment of burn syndactyly. Plastic and Reconstructive Surgery 57: 167–171

MacLeod A M, O'Brien B McC, Morrison W A 1985 Microvascular free flaps. In: Tubiana R (ed) The hand, Vol. II. Saunders, Philadelphia

Marin-Braun F, Merle M, Foucher G 1988 Le lambeau cerf-volant. Annales de Chirurgie de la Main 7: 147–150

Maruyama Y 1990 The reverse dorsal metacarpal flap. British Journal of Plastic Surgery 43: 24–27

Masquelet A C, Penteado C V 1987 Le lambeau interosseux postérieur. Annales de Chirurgie de la Main 6: 131–139

Matthews R N, Morgan B D G 1987 Multiple seagull flaps for digital contractures in electrical burns. British Journal of Plastic Surgery 40: 47–51

Mir y Mir L 1973 The six-flap Z-plasty. Plastic and Reconstructive Surgery 52: 625–628

Miura T 1979 Use of paired abdominal flaps for release of adduction contractures of the thumb. Plastic and Reconstructive Surgery 63: 242–244

Moberg E 1964 Aspects of sensation in reconstructive surgery of the upper extremity. Journal of Bone and Joint Surgery 46A: 817–825

Monks G H 1898 The restoration of a lower eyelid by a new method. Boston Medical and Surgical Journal 139: 385–387

Mustardé J C 1963 Epicanthus and telecanthus. British Journal of Plastic Surgery 16: 346–356

Mutz S B 1972 Thumb web contracture. Hand 4: 236–246

Oberlin C, Le Quang C 1985 Etude anatomique de la vascularisation du lambeau en drapeau. Annales de Chirurgie de la Main 4: 169–174

Oberlin C, Sarcy J J, Alnot J Y 1988 Apport artériel cutané de la main. Application à la réalisation des lambeaux en îlot. Annales de Chirurgie de la Main 7: 122–125

Ostrowski D M, Feagin C A, Gould J S 1991 A three-flap web-plasty for release of short congenital syndactyly and dorsal adduction contracture. Journal of Hand Surgery 16 A: 634–641

Pensler J M, Steward R, Lewis S R, Herndon D N 1988 Reconstruction of the burned palm: full-thickness versus split-thickness skin grafts – long-term follow-up. Plastic and Reconstructive Surgery 81: 46–49

Quaba A A, Davison P M 1990 The distally based dorsal hand flap. British Journal of Plastic Surgery 43: 28–39

Riordan D C, cited by Lister G D, Milward T M 1976 Skin contracture of the first web space. Transactions of the Sixth International Congress of Plastic and Reconstructive Surgery, Paris, August 1975

Rousso M 1975 Brûlures dorsales graves de la main. Réconstruction de la commissure. Technique à cinq lambeaux. 1er partie. Le premiére commissure. Annales de Chirurgie 29: 475–479

Sandzén S C 1982 Dorsal pedicle flap for resurfacing a moderate thumb–index web contracture release. Journal of Hand Surgery 7: 21–24

Scheker L R, Lister G D, Wolff T W 1988 The lateral arm free flap in release severe contracture of the first web space. Journal of Hand Surgery 13B: 1946–1950

Shaw D T, Li C S, Richey D G, Nahigian S H 1972 Interdigital butterfly flap (the double opposing Z-plasty). Handchirurgie 4: 41–43

Shaw D T, Li C S, Richey D G, Nahigian S H 1973 Interdigital butterfly flap in the hand (the double-opposing Z-plasty). Journal of Bone and Joint Surgery 55: 1677–1679

Small J O, Brennen M D 1988 The first dorsal metacarpal artery neurovascular island flap. Journal of Hand Surgery 13B: 136–145

Small J O, Brennen M D 1990 The second dorsal metacarpal artery neurovascular island flap. British Journal of Plastic Surgery 43: 17–23

Smith P J, Harrison S H 1982 The 'seagull' flap for syndactyly. British Journal of Plastic Surgery 35: 390–393

Spinner M 1969 Fashioned transpositional flap for soft tissue adduction contracture of the thumb. Plastic and Reconstructive Surgery 44: 345–348

Strauch B 1975 Dorsal thumb flap for release of adduction contracture of the first web space. Bulletin of the Hospital for Joint Diseases XXXVI: 34–39

Strickland J W 1982 Reconstruction of the contracted first web space. In: Strickland J W, Steichen J B (eds) Difficult problems in hand surgery. C.V. Mosby, Saint Louis

Tajima T 1985 Classification of thumb hypoplasia. Hand Clinics 1: 577–594

Tanzer R C 1948 Correction of interdigital burn contractures of the hand. Plastic and Recontructive Surgery 3: 434–438

Teich-Alasia S, Barberis M L 1972 The value of the 'cross-arm' flap in reconstructive surgery of the hand. Chirurgia Plastica (Berlin) 1: 134–144

Thomine J-M 1971 Surgical treatment of post-traumatic

retraction of the first interdigital commissure (in French and English). In: Vilain R (ed) Les traumatismes ostéo-articulaires de la main. Monographies du Groupe d'Etude de la Main No. 4. L'Expansion Scientifique Française, Paris

Thomine J-M 1985 Stiffness of the trapeziometacarpal joint and post-traumatic retraction of the first web space. In: Tubiana R (ed) The hand, Vol II Saunders, Philadelphia

Tubiana R 1985 Skin flaps. In: Tubiana R (ed) The hand, Vol. II. Saunders, Philadelphia

Tubiana R, Duparc J 1961 Restoration of sensibility in the hand by neurovascular skin island transfer. Journal of Bone and Joint Surgery 43B: 474–480

Tubiana R, Duparc J, Moreau C 1960 Restauration de la sensibilité au niveau de la main par transfert d'un transplant cutané hétéro-digital muni de son pédicule vasculo-nerveux. Revue de Chirurgie Orthopedique 46: 163–178

Vilain R 1952 Technique élémentaire de réparation des pertes de substance cutanée des doigts. Semaine des Hôpitaux de Paris 28: 1223–1229

Vilain R, Dupuis J F 1973 Use of the flag flap for coverage of a small area on a finger or the palm. 20 years' experience. Plastic and Reconstructive Surgery 51: 397–401

Wintsch K, Schneider K, Ganzoni N 1971 Die Korrektur der Adduktionskontraktur des Daumens. Handchirurgie 3: 71–76

Woolf R M, Broadbent T R 1972 The four-flap Z-plasty. Plastic and Reconstructive Surgery 49: 48–51

Yeschua R, Wexler M R, Neuman Z 1977 Cross-arm triangular flaps for correction of adduction contracture of the first web space in the hand. Case report. Plastic and Reconstructive Surgery 59: 859–861

Zancolli E A, Angrigiani C 1988 Posterior interosseous island forearm flap. Journal of Hand Surgery 13B: 130–135

15 Therapeutic approach in fingertip injuries

Loss of a fingertip can render an otherwise normal finger useless by causing its functional exclusion from the normal activities of the hand. The fingertip pulp plays a fundamental role in grip by virtue of its specialized covering. Pulp skin is thick – not only the keratinized epidermal part, but also the dermis, which has deep dermal papillae. It does not bear follicles, but on histological examination is seen to contain, besides the sweat glands, numerous sensory endings: Merkel's disks, Meissner's corpuscles and Vater-Pacini corpuscles. Jabaley et al (1976) have, however, shown that the density of these nerve endings is not proportional to the quality of the sensory discrimination: discussion also remains open as to whether these endings are simply reinnervated, or newly created, following proximal damage to the afferent nerve.

This cutaneous covering is firmly fixed to the skeleton of the distal phalanx by fibrous expansions which subdivide the pulp, whilst lateral fixation is furnished by the lateral ligament of the distal phalanx under which runs the blood and nerve supply to the nail. The nail plays an important part in stabilizing the pulp and enhancing the quality of sensation by its counter-pressure. A unique construction thus confers on the pulp a firm base and reduced mobility. This, associated with an antislip surface kept moist by sweat glands, together with numerous nerve endings enabling sophisticated discrimination, gives the pulp its exceptional properties in grip, namely finesse, force and precision; and in touch, heat and pain sensibility.

It can easily be imagined what problems might be posed in reconstructing a substantial loss of pulp, charged as it is with giving quasi-visual information to the central cerebral 'computer'. In practice there are two problems, closely interlinked. These are sensibility and/or pain due to hypersensitivity. When use returns to an injured finger, cerebral reintegration is spontaneous. When, however, pain or mediocrity of sensory quality prevent normal use, especially with an isolated finger injury, this leads to cerebral exclusion. The index is particularly prone to this. Such a state of affairs may become entrenched, and the hypersensitivity is not particularly amenable to sensory treatment. It must be stressed that in the immediate aftermath of a local plastic operation on a finger, hypersensitivity is a frequent but temporary phenomenon. Simple tapping of the end, and rubbing with a fabric of increasing roughness, will condition the new nerve endings and improve the mechanical characteristics of the new skin covering and its surrounding borders of scar tissue. As for sensation, one of the greatest advances in recent years has been sensory reeducation following nerve injury. Wynn Parry and Salter (1976) and Dellon (1981) have for many years insisted on the importance of this reeducation, firstly to reduce the initial hyperaesthesia, and secondly to improve sensory discrimination.

METHODS

First of all those cases where the amputated fragment of fingertip is usable must be distinguished from those where it is not. If the fragment is usable there is no doubt that the best treatment remains replantation (Foucher et al 1981b) even in very distal cases, distal to the distal interphalangeal joint. The authors have reviewed 53 very distal replantations in 51 patients, of which 28 were treated as day cases, the others being hospitalized for a mean of 5.3 days. In the absence of a venous repair, leeches were used with success in 72.7%. In successful cases, the mean time off work was 73 days, as opposed to 87 days in cases of failure. The mean discrimination on two-point testing in successful cases was 9.5 mm. The advantages of this replantation appear to be evident:

1. The operation is simple and quick (mean time 75 minutes) because there is no need to repair any tendons, and osteosynthesis by a single axial K-wire is very simple.
2. Immediate mobilization of the proximal interphalangeal joint is allowed.
3. Sensory recovery is fast (mean 4.5 months)
4. It is a good means of preventing painful distal neuromas, which remain one of the great problems of distal amputations.
5. The cosmetic aspect is good because the nail is conserved.

Even if the skeleton is not usable it is still possible to fashion a free pulp flap taken from the fragment and to revascularize and neurotize it at the level of the distal cut, which the authors have done in six cases.

If no vessels can be found on microscopic examination of the fragment, simple reposition remains an alternative. Douglas (1959) defined its limits: clean section in a young patient seen immediately after the accident. This method has shown itself to be unreliable, however, with 5 complete failures out of 11 attempts in the authors' experience. This is the reason why we now prefer a modification in which the amputated fingertip is replaced and the palmar skin segment of it immediately excised, being replaced by a local flap advanced from the same finger. This technique enables a good blood supply to be brought to the distal replaced fragment, which at this point consists only of bone and nailbed, and at the same time to obtain a sensitive palmar skin covering for the pulp. In eight cases the authors have only had one failure, but healing is slow, the nailbed passing through a phase of mummification. If the distal fragment is not usable it can be

regarded as a 'finger bank' (Foucher et al 1980b, 1986), in other words a finger which would have to be sacrificed anyway for vital or functional reasons, but in which certain tissue elements could be used either as an island flap or as a free flap. For example, it is thus possible to use the palmar skin of an index finger which is not worth retaining due to severe bony injury or loss, either as an island flap if the arterial supply is intact (three cases), or as a free flap (two cases). Sometimes in distal amputation of the thumb a composite transfer can be performed using components (skin, bone, nailbed, nail complex) belonging to a finger bank. In cases of crush injury to the hand, these extensive dissections are contraindicated and it is preferable to 'stock' the fragment in situ for secondary reconstruction (three cases). This two-stage technique is always more delicate than the immediate transfer of an 'on-top plasty', which the authors have performed six times as a one-stage procedure in an acute injury. A good indication for these emergency transfers is when there has been an extensive loss of dorsal skin and bone, especially affecting the proximal interphalangeal joint where 'stocking' of the finger is dubious and where the transfer will permit excellent cosmetic results to be obtained thanks to the persistence of the nail. In the absence of recoverable tissues, it may be necessary to resort to the classic methods, namely, shortening, healing by secondary intention, local flaps, regional flaps or remote flaps. The authors believe that shortening of the skeleton is less and less indicated. It is far preferable to advance a local flap, which will avoid a distal scar by having a more dorsal scar together with dorsal translocation of the ends of the digital nerves where they are less subject to painful stimulation. This method thus permits better skin cover to be brought to the distal part of a mutilated finger.

One must not underestimate the marvellous possibility offered by nature of delayed healing which is not spontaneous but rather 'directed'. A distal loss of substance can be spontaneously filled in by granulation tissue. Vilain (1954), in France, showed more than 20 years ago that granulation tissue is amenable to stimulation by a simple 'tulle gras' dressing, and when the bulk of the pulp has reconstituted he then facilitated reepithelialization by anti-inflammatory dressings based on topical corticosteroids. Epithelialization takes place by the advance of cells from the wound edges, and at the same time by contraction of the margins of the wound; this has the effect of pulling in healthy tissue from around the margins. This healing by secondary intention is not limited by the age of the patient, although in young people the process is more rapid. Nor is it limited by the area of loss of substance, but by depth, and the method is not recommended when bone or tendon is exposed. It must be added that this method is relatively slow, as the authors' series of 77 cases treated by this method over a period of 12 months showed: healing took 36 days on average, and the time off work was 58 days due to the temporary but disabling hypersensitivity of the regenerated fingertip.

Among other methods, only local flaps, hetero-digital palmar island flaps and skin taken from the level of the palm or from the toes, allow skin to be brought in whose texture and structure are comparable with those of recipient site.

There are numerous local flaps, but the V-Y flaps of Kutler (1947) and those of Tranquilli-Leali (1935) and Atasoy et al (1970) are the best known (Fig. 15.1). The authors have abandoned the flap of Kutler in favour of the second type, and after raising the flap it is fixed distally to the skeleton and not to the nailbed, so as to avoid any traction – a factor known to cause the development of a claw nail. In addition the V-Y plasty is not closed, so as to avoid decreasing the transverse diameter of the finger and hence possibly compressing the pedicles of the flap. For a larger and oblique loss of substance the Hueston (1966) flap is used. This is an L-shape, and classically the neurovascular pedicle lying under the long branch of the L is not included in the flap; this gives skin cover of rather mediocre sensibility. In fact both bundles can be included in the flap, thus limiting the advancement. The proximal loss of substance can be left to heal spontaneously or be covered by a partial-thickness skin graft. The authors prefer to use a triangular flap taken from the side of the finger, whose advancement allows primary closure of the defect (Foucher et al 1985).

The flap of Moberg (Moberg 1964), which was one of the first to be described, is used only in the thumb where the vascularization of the dorsal skin is independent. This flap is cut from the entire palmar surface of the remaining thumb and, with the aid of flexion of the interphalangeal joint,

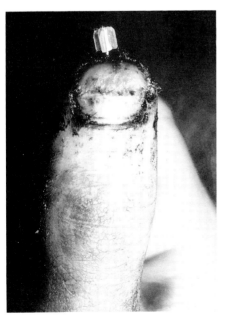

A

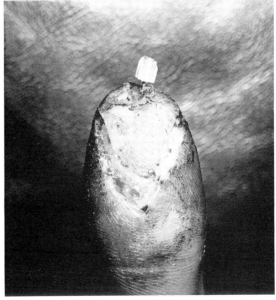

B

Fig. 15.1A, B Distal fixation of a volar V-Y island flap (Tranquilli-Leali) using a needle in the distal phalanx. The nailbed is lengthened with a split-skin graft from the hypothenar eminence.

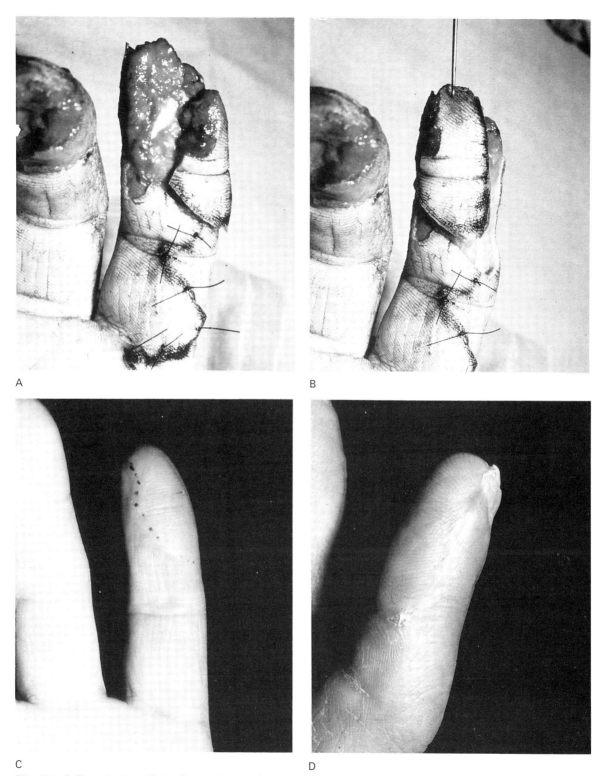

A

B

C

D

Fig. 15.2 A Extensive loss of index finger pulp, exposing bone and tendon. A homodigital advancement flap has been raised.
B Advancement of the flap to reach the fingertip. **C, D** The final result at 3 months.

allows distal cover. Snow (1967) has described the use of this flap in the other fingers, but the risk of necrosis of the dorsal skin is significant unless one locates and preserves the dorsal branches of the digital arteries at the level of the proximal phalanx.

The O'Brien flap (O'Brien 1968) is a bipedicled island flap which allows skin advancement distally. This skin is of excellent quality for obtaining good sensibility in the new fingertip. In this case also, rather than rely on healing by secondary intention or a split-skin graft to cover the defect left proximally by advancement of the flap, the authors prefer to swing two little triangular flaps over the defect, which give an excellent bed for the neurovascular pedicles and avoid late loss of the sensory recovery.

The most recently described local flap, the unipedicled homodigital flap (Venkataswami and Subramaniam 1980, Mouchet & Gilbert 1982), allows coverage of loss due to amputation. A substantial advancement of this island flap is possible by dissecting the neurovascular pedicle down to the palm. The most easy advancement, and also the greatest in magnitude, is obtained in the index finger thanks to the freeing of the pedicle at the level of the neck of the second metacarpal, followed by its medialization. The finger is kept in flexion at the level of the metacarpophalangeal joint for 10 days, with only slight flexion of the proximal interphalangeal joint. A dynamic extension splint is necessary after 10 days, as in the authors' 70 cases a fixed flexion deficit of the proximal interphalangeal joint was noted (mean 7° in 13%) (Fig. 15.2).

Particularly difficult problems of sensibility are often solved by using the palmar heterodigital island flaps of Littler (1956). The problem of sensibility is quite complex and the tests in use today remain largely academic; it is the utilization of the finger which is the most important factor, and it is not rare to see a flap which seems to possess a perfect two-point discrimination nevertheless being excluded from daily use. This is sometimes the case in the heterodigital flaps of Littler which can bring normal two-point discrimination to a thumb but impair the use of the thumb due to cerebral misrepresentation. In certain cases it is preferable to section the nerve and to suture it to the distal end of the proximal stump of the recipient-site nerve (De Coninck 1975, Foucher et al 1981c). The quality of sensation then becomes inferior to what it was previously, but the utilization is better. It is important to prevent a distal neuroma on the proximal end of the donor nerve by cutting it well down in the palm and translocating it dorsally in the interosseous space, as proposed by Littler in the treatment of neuromas.

Palmar skin can be also used in the form of thenar flaps, as modified by Melone et al (1982). These flaps raised at the base of the thumb enable significant losses of substance to be filled, but the results from the sensory point of view have led the authors to use them only for the ring and middle fingers. The modifications suggested by Melone avoid hypersensibility at the donor site and too much flexion at the proximal interphalangeal joint. The authors cut the pedicle at about the 12th day in order to avoid adverse sequelae in the recipient finger, and immediately use dynamic extension splintage in order to straighten the finger once more. On the other hand the final trimming and adjustment of the flap on a recipient finger is not performed until after the third week. This adjustment is not always necessary, as delayed secondary healing often causes a retraction which assures an excellent result without the need for further surgical procedure.

Different techniques have been described for taking skin from the toes. These may be composite grafts such as those described by Maquieira and McCash. The authors only use the technique of McCash (1959) in children, in whom it has given excellent results. The pulp of the third toe is taken, together with the underlying fat, and carefully sutured to the recipient site. This method has not been successful in the adult patient, and the authors have observed so many failures (7 out of 9) that they have now abandoned it. McCash reported excellent results as regards sensibility, but the authors have found it difficult to test in our young patients.

The technique of Maquieira (1974) consists of taking pulp from the toe and defatting it very carefully, preserving the digital branches. This composite graft, consisting of skin and nerve but not fat, is then transferred to the recipient site where the nerve is sutured end-to-end and the grafts put in place. This is a tedious technique and does not seem to offer any advantage over microsurgical techniques, whose reliability appears to be better.

Free vascularized pulp transfers from the toes (Buncke & Rose 1979, Foucher et al 1980a, 1981a, Logan et al 1985) are available thanks to the advent of microsurgical techniques. The artery, vein and nerve are identified, harvested with the pulp and then sutured to their counterparts at the receiver site. The advantage of this technique is that it allows the inclusion of vascularized bone, nailbed, or the whole nail complex. A clear advantage has been noted in vascularized bone grafts in these distal situations as opposed to non-vascularized grafts, which have a tendency to resorb, however good the vascularization of the adjacent soft tissues (Foucher 1982). Skin grafts have frequently been recommended for covering loss of substance in the distal parts of the finger, but they only replace the surface and do not address the problem of the loss of tissue volume and cushioning. The majority of good results are explained by retraction, which is helped by the mobility of the underlying tissues.

Recovery of sensibility in the graft has been studied by numerous authors. Charvat and Smahal (1965) showed in the rat that nerve regeneration begins from the third and fourth days, with penetration into the graft by the eighth day, either in the empty neural tubes or in the tissues themselves. Fitzgerald (1967) did not show any nervous response for the second week, and showed that the majority of fibres grew into the empty nerve sheaths, with the final result corresponding to their density. Kadanoff (Moberg 1964) studying 15 human grafts, found regrowth of the nerves along the vessels and partially into the graft itself, underlining the infrequency of regeneration for specific nerve endings. Ponten (1960), studying different types of sensibility, found a more than adequate recovery in full-thickness skin grafts which had taken completely, allowing the acquisition of a sensibility identical to that of the donor site. Many other authors have stressed that, depending on the adaptation after functional use, or on sensory reeducation, sensory performances superior to those of the donor site are possible (Waris 1978, Wynn Parry & Salter 1976, Dellon 1981). This particularly interesting

point was underlined by Matev, who reviewed palmar grafts performed in children from 2 to 5 years of age. When seen at age 13–19, these grafts showed normal sensibility, including two-point discrimination. All the authors stressed the absence on histological examination of reinnervation of specific receptors. What then can be concluded on the practical level from these findings in the literature? Grafts give good results as regards sensibility when they are performed in children, when the skin is thick, when the donor site is rich in sensory endings, and when the functional utilization is good. On the other hand, in the adult, the sensory result is rather poor (Moberg 1964, Mannerfelt 1962, Terzis 1976).

Bearing in mind the characteristics of palmar skin, it is clear that the dorsal skin – fine, supple, elastic and hair-bearing – cannot bring the same mechanical and sensory qualities to the palmar surface when used as a cross-finger flap. However, the results observed by Beasley (1969) are of interest: in about 100 cases he observed a mean two-point discrimination of 9 mm. Certain authors, including Berger and Meissl (1975), have proposed an improvement in the sensibility of cross-finger flaps by the anastomosis of dorsal nerves at the level of the recipient site.

It is equally evident that the majority of distant flaps, even if they do not bring bulk in their underflying fatty tissue (often too abundant), do not resolve the basic problems of sensibility and the stability necessary in grip. As has been seen, they find a rare indication in extensive multidigital huge skin loss, and the flap graft of Colson (1970) appears to be the best suited for this purpose.

INDICATIONS

It is difficult to make a formal plan of the different techniques and their indications, since they will depend on a number of factors. Certain of these will relate to the surgeon, others to the patient, and others (among them the most important) to the type of trauma. It must first of all be established that the factor relating to the surgeon is his competence. It is catastrophic to lose a local flap, because this considerably aggravates the lesions and makes their treatment more difficult.

It is preferable in the light of limited experience to opt for delayed healing or a skin graft, planning a plastic procedure as secondary repair.

The factors relating to the patient equally merit attention. They relate to age, sex, associated diseases and the professional occupation and leisure pursuits of the patient. The needs of a manual worker, where the skin covering has an essentially protective role, cannot be compared with those of a watchmaker whose fine manipulation requires an excellent touch sensation. There can be some very sophisticated indications, such as the free transfer of part of the big toe in order to reconstruct a good quality pulp and nail. Leisure activities such as playing a musical instrument can lead the surgeon to modify his choice of procedure. In such cases the number of affected fingers, their length, mobility and sensibility play an important role. The cosmetic appearance, where the role of the nail is important, should not be neglected in women and one can opt for conservation even of the proximal one-third of the nailbed. Later on, a proximal nail shifting (Verdan 1978) with advancement of a volar flap may reduce the 'parrot beak' deformity. Equally the needs of the patient who runs a small business or farm, and who wants to return as fast as possible to his activity without undergoing an ambitious programme of reconstruction or rehabilitation, must be borne in mind. The age of the patient might perhaps appear to be the most important factor, but its limits are rather fluid. Ages can be thought of as two groups: first a 'vascular' age for operations such as island flaps, and a 'nervous age', over which sensory recovery after nerve suture will always be insufficient. This nervous age is the important consideration in free pulp transfer, not for the survival of the pulp, but for the functional result of the nerve suture, and it is the authors' opinion that indications for such surgery cannot apply to patients much over 35 years.

Existing medical conditions must also be borne in mind, and this is not always easy in an emergency. The diabetic will generally inform the surgeon, but a homodigital island advancement flap was lost in a patient aged 37 years who had Raynaud's syndrome, but who did not think it necessary to mention this in summertime when he was free of symptoms.

It must, however, be underlined that it is the factors related to the injury itself which remain the most important, notably the type of trauma, the ray affected, the extent and the obliquity of the loss of substance, and the presence or absence of recoverable and usable tissues in the neighbourhood. As regards the type of injury, frostbite, crush injury and heavy contamination are contraindications to primary treatment by a flap. Crushing makes it difficult to define the limits of tissue loss, and adds an 'at risk' zone to the real loss. Significant contamination gives rise to real risk during any extensive dissection. Avulsion is a particular mechanism which has an important effect as regards the nerve tissue, and is a contraindication to the use of a free pulp transfer or a nerve anastomosis in a heterodigital island flap, because of the proximal extent of the nerve lesions. One cannot apportion equal importance to the radial pulp of the index and the ulnar pulp of the ring finger. This is the reason why indications vary according to the affected ray and pulp. The authors no longer practise skin grafts, cross-finger flaps or thenar flaps for the thumb and the index, but reserve them for injuries to the third, fourth or fifth rays. In lesions of the index and of the thumb, the authors favour local flaps, homodigital and heterodigital island flaps and even sophisticated techniques such as 'custom-made' reconstructions from the toes. When several long fingers are affected, a distant flap may be needed in the first instance and in this case the preference is for the Colson flap graft. When the index is affected by the lesion the authors will proceed at a second stage to restoring sensibility to the radial side either by a homodigital island advancement flap, heterodigital island flap, or microsurgical free pulp transfer.

Lastly, three factors are important: the extent of the loss of substance, its obliquity, and the presence or absence of usable tissues in the neighbourhood. It must yet again be stressed that if the patient's age lends itself, the best treatment for amputations, even very distal ones, is replantation of the affected part. The authors have already mentioned their results which appear highly satisfactory in young subjects (Fig. 15.3).

The extent and the obliquity are two very important factors in the choice of technique. In

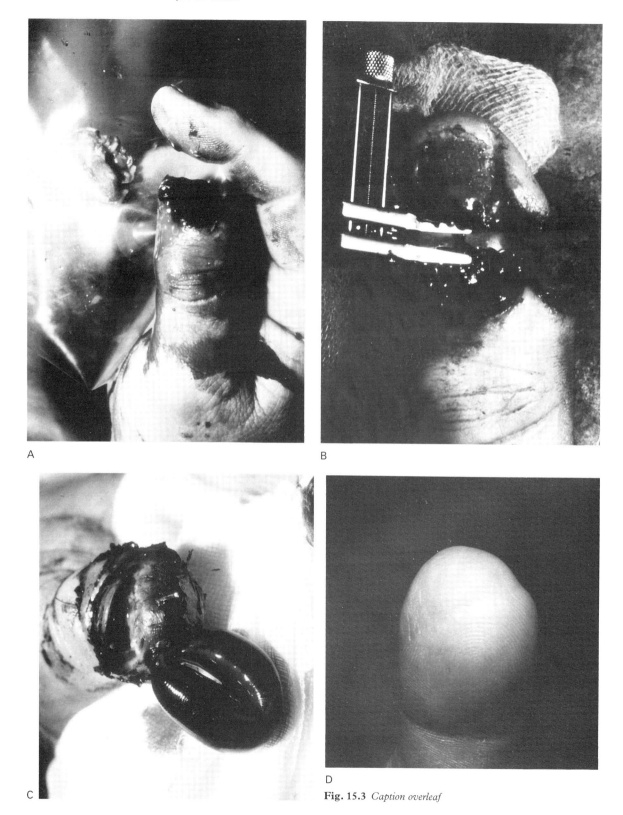

A

B

C

D

Fig. 15.3 *Caption overleaf*

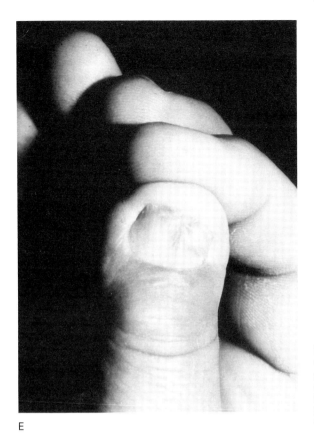

E

Fig. 15.3 A Amputation of the tip of the thumb in a patient whose other hand has been amputated. **B** For this distal replantation an artery was anastomosed through the nailbed using a dorsal approach. **C** No venous repair was performed, but leeches were used for 5 days to avoid venous congestion. **D, E** The final result at 6 months. Two-point discrimination was 8 mm.

practice there are many local flaps, but their advancement is variable and the decision will depend then on the obliquity and the loss of substance. For example, hemipulp loss on the radial side of the index would indicate either an 'exchange' island flap of Littler, favouring the more important pulp in covering the distal skeleton, or a Hueston flap, of which the major drawback is the bringing distally of moderately insensitive skin covering, since it is separated from one digital nerve. A transverse section can usually be covered by a volar V-Y advancement (Tranquilli-Leali–Atasoy) flap which the authors prefer to the lateral V-Y (Kutler) flap. The scope for advancement of these flaps, however, remains limited. In our experience (Foucher et al 1986), it is a mean of 5 mm in a series of 257 Atasoy flaps and 8 mm in a series of 195 Hueston flaps.

When the obliquity of palmar slope is greater the flap of Moberg can be used in the thumb, giving a mean advancement of 9 mm. For the longer fingers the authors do not use the technique of Snow (1967), but prefer the bipedicled island flap of O'Brien (1968), of which the mean advancement in their 34 cases was 11 mm. In large palmar losses of skin the best advancement is obtained by a monopedicled island flap (mean advancement 12 mm, maximum 20 mm). When a large loss of substance in an oblique amputation affects the middle, ring or little fingers, the cross-finger flap appears to to be a possibility. The authors have used 49 cross-finger flaps, 32 according to the classic technique, 8 from a 'finger bank' and 9 remaining cases with reinnervation (Adamson et al 1967, Gaul 1969, Brailliar & Horner 1969), or as de-epithelialized flaps as described by Pakiam (1978), and adapted by Atasoy (1982).

Contrary to what has been found by Beasley (1969), the authors' results have not been encouraging from the point of view of two-point discrimination, which was more than 12 mm in the majority of their cases, except in two very young subjects where it was found to be 9 mm. In the thumb we have attempted to improve the sensibility of these cross-finger flaps by using the technique described by Brailliar (1969), Gaul (1969) and Adamson et al (1967) in subjects more than 40 years old. In the first stage the cross-finger flap was made from the dorsal part of the index, with translocation of the radial nerve and its branches to the recipient site. For subjects between 30 and 40 years old the authors prefer to use the kite flap (Foucher & Braun 1979), which allows the transfer of the sensitive skin surface in one stage as an island flap. Before the age of 30 preference goes to the Littler (1956) heterodigital flap, which gives a better performance with or without nerve repair at the recipient site. It is only in huge losses of substance in oblique amputations of the index and thumb in young patients that the authors resort to free vascularized partial toe transfer. Another indication involves the composite loss of substance where it is necessary to bring, besides pulp, a fragment of vascularized bone and a nailbed flap to support the nail. The results in these pulp transfers are encouraging. In 38 operations performed by the authors, the mean age was 23 years;

23 of these transfers were performed on the thumb, the others having been performed on the index or on the middle finger (in the absence of the index). There were two failures and with a mean follow-up of 39 months the two-point discrimination was 11 mm, and moving two-point discrimination 9 mm. Five cases, however, did show discrimination greater than 15 mm. In three of these cases the index was excluded from fine touch but was utilized in power grip.

One of the important points which has not yet been not mentioned is frequent cold intolerance at the donor site. This intolerance decreases after two winters but, contrary to what is normally stated, does not disappear completely even 10 years after the operation.

In conclusion, the loss of pulp substance is a frequent injury whose seriousness is underestimated. Sometimes neglected, often treated by general practitioners or general surgeons, this injury can give rise to prolonged absence from work and even to permanent disability. The large number of available methods gives hand surgeons the opportunity to choose, in each case, the simplest technique that will bring about the best result.

REFERENCES

Adamson J E, Horton C E, Crawford H H 1967 Sensory rehabilitation of the injured thumb. Plastic and Reconstructive Surgery 40: 53–57
Atasoy E 1982 The reversed cross-finger subcutaneous flap. Journal of Hand Surgery 7: 481–483
Atasoy E, Ioakimidis E, Kasdan M L et al 1970 Reconstruction of the amputated finger tip with a triangular volar flap. Journal of Bone and Joint Surgery 52A: 921–926
Beasley R W 1969 Reconstruction of amputated fingertips. Plastic and Reconstructive Surgery 44: 349–352
Berger A, Meissl G 1975 Innervated skin grafts and flaps for restoration of sensation to anaesthetic areas. Chirurgia Plastica 3: 33-37
Brailliar F, Horner R L 1969 Sensory cross-finger pedicle graft. Journal of Bone and Joint Surgery 51A: 1264–1268
Buncke H J, Rose E H 1979 Free toe-to-finger tip neurovascular flaps. Plastic and Reconstructive Surgery 63: 607–612
Charvat Z, Smahel J 1965 Reinnervation of a free skin autograft. Acta Chirurgica, Orthopedica, Traumatologica. Technica. 32: 531-536
Colson P 1970 Le lambeau dermo-épidermique. Chirurgie 96: 639–643
De Coninck A 1975 Transplantation hétéro-digitale avec reinnervation locale. Acta Orthopedica Belgica 41: 170–176

Dellon A L 1981 Evaluation of sensibility and reeducation of sensation in the hand. Williams & Wilkins, Baltimore and London
Douglas B 1959 Successful replacement of completely avulsed portions of fingers as composite grafts. Plastic and Reconstructive Surgery 23: 213-225
Fitzgerald M J T 1967 Innervation of skin grafts. Surgery, Gynecology and Obstetrics 124: 808–812
Foucher G 1982 Indications du transfert osseux vascularisé en chirurgie de la main. Revule de Chirurgie Orthopédique 68: Suppl. II 38–39
Foucher G, Braun J B 1979 A new island flap transfer from the dorsum of the index to the thumb. Plastic and Reconstructive Surgery 63: 344–349
Foucher G, Braun F M, Merle M, Michon J 1980b Le doigt 'banque' en traumatologie de la main. Annales de Chirurgie 34: 693–698
Foucher G, Braun F M, Merle M, Michon J 1981a Les problémes techniques et les indications des transferts de pulpe d'orteil. Annales de Chirurgie Plastique 26: 2–7
Foucher G, Braun F M, Merle M, Michon J 1981c La technique du debranchement–rebranchement' du lambeau en ilot pedicule. Annales de Chirurgie 35: 301–303
Foucher G, Henderson H R, Maneaud M et al 1981b Distal digital replantation: one of the best indications for

microsurgery. International Journal of Microsurgery 3: 263–270

Foucher G, Merle M, Michon J 1986 Les amputations digitales distales: de la cicatrisation dirigée au transfert microchirurgical de pulpe d'orteil. Chirurgie 112: 727–735

Foucher G, Merle M, Maneaud M, Michon J 1980a Microsurgical free partial toe transfer in hand reconstruction. Plastic and Reconstructive Surgery 65: 616–627

Foucher G, Sibilly A, Merle M, Michon J 1985b Le lambeau de Hueston dans les recouvrements de pertes de substance distale du pouce. Annales de Chirurgie de la Main 4: 239–241

Gaul J S 1969 Radial-innervated cross-finger flap from index to provide sensory pulp to injured thumb. Journal of Bone and Joint Surgery 51A: 1257–1263

Hueston J 1966 Local flap repair of fingertip injuries. Plastic and Reconstructive Surgery 37: 349–350

Jabaley M E, Burns J A, Orcutt B S, Bryant W M 1976 Comparison of histologic and functional recovery after peripheral nerve repair. Journal of Hand Surgery 1: 119–130

Kutler W 1947 A new method for fingertip amputations. Journal of the American Medical Association 133: 23–30

Littler J W 1956 Neurovascular pedicle transfer of tissue in reconstructive surgery of the hand. Journal of Bone and Joint Surgery 38A: 917

Logan A, Elliot D, Foucher G 1985 Free toe pulp transfer to restore traumatic digital pulp loss. British Journal of Plastic Surgery 38: 497–500

McCash C R 1959 The pulp free graft in finger tip repair. British Journal of Plastic Surgery 11: 322–326

Maquieira N O 1974 An innervated full-thickness skin graft to restore sensibility to fingertips and heels. Plastic and Reconstructive Surgery 53: 568–575

Mannerfeldt L 1962 Evaluation of functional sensation of skin grafts in the hand area. British Journal of Plastic Surgery 15: 136–154

Melone C P, Beasley R W, Crastens J H 1982 The thenar flap – an analysis of its use in 150 cases. Journal of Hand Surgery 7: 291–297

Moberg E 1964 Aspect of sensation in reconstructive surgery of the upper extremity. Journal of Bone and Joint Surgery 46: 817–825

Mouchet A, Gilbert A 1982 Couverture des amputations distales des doigts par lambeau neurovasculaire homodigital en ilot. Annales de Chirurgie de la Main 1: 180–182

O'Brien B McC 1968 Neurovascular island pedicle flaps for terminal amputations and digital scars. Journal of Bone and Joint Surgery 21: 258–261

Pakiam I A 1978 The reversed dermis flap. British Journal of Plastic Surgery 31: 131–135

Ponten B 1960 Grafted skin: observations on innervation and other qualities. Acta Chirurgia Scandinavica, Supplement, 78: 257–268

Snow J W 1967 The use of a volar flap for repair of fingertip amputations: a preliminary report. Plastic and Reconstructive Surgery 40: 163–168

Terzis J K 1976 Functional aspects of reinnervation of free skin grafts. Plastic and Reconstructive Surgery 58: 142–153

Tranquilli-Leali E 1935 Riconstruzione dell'apice delle falange ungeali mediante autoplastica volare. Infort. Traum. Lavoro 1: 186–193

Venkataswami R, Subramanian N 1980 Oblique triangular flap: a new method of repair for oblique amputations of the fingertip and thumb. Plastic and Reconstructive Surgery 66: 296–299

Verdan C 1978 Chirurgie plastique de l'ongle en griffe. Monographie du GEM. L'Expansion

Vilain R 1954 Les pertes de substance cutanée des doigts et leur traitement (à propos de 100 observations). Annales de Chirurgie 4: 197-212

Waris T 1978 Reinnervation of free skin autografts in the rat. Scandinavian Journal of Plastic and Reconstructive Surgery 12: 85–93

Wynn Parry C B, Salter M 1976 Sensory reeducation after median nerve lesions. Hand 8: 250–255

16 Skin cover in burns

Burn injuries to the hand are common. In Tord Skoog's survey 'The Surgical Treatment of Burns' (Skoog, 1963) 262 of 789 patients admitted to the burns unit during 19 years had one or both hands affected. Altogether 384 hands were treated, most of which had full-thickness burns. During the same period 625 of 1622 less severe burns were treated as outpatients with superficially burned hands. This incidence rate has not changed over the years in the authers' burns unit: still just over one-third have hand burns.

The principles of treatment, however, have changed. Before 1978 burns were treated conservatively until the extent of the coagulation process could be determined. Removal of the slough was generally delayed until at least 14 days after injury. Following debridement the wound was covered by split-skin grafts either immediately or 1–2 days later, if bleeding was not easily controlled. Elevation and active motion were used to diminish swelling, and the hand was splinted in a functional position between sessions of physiotherapy. However the pain during the period before skin cover was complete often made training difficult.

Since 1978 all full-thickness and deep dermal burns of the hand have been excised primarily during the first or second day after injury, and grafted according to Jackson et al (1960) and Janzekovic (1968, 1970). Pressure gloves are used after healing to reduce scar hypertrophy.

PRIMARY EXCISION OF BURNS IN THE HAND

Diagnosis

Deep dermal burns are characterized by a white to

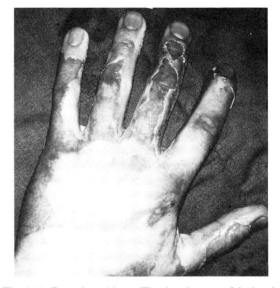

Fig. 16.1 Deep dermal burn. The dorsal aspect of the hand is white, without capillary circulation and pain sensation. The fingers are red owing to erythrocyte haemolysis.

red-brown surface, reduced or absent capillary circulation and impaired pain sensation or complete anaesthesia. In the case of deep dermal burns with a white surface, reduced capillary circulation and impaired pain sensation, a second examination is recommended after 24 hours (Fig. 16.1). Full-thickness burns are characterized by a yellow-grey or dark brown surface, with no capillary circulation and complete anaesthesia.

The ideal time for primary excision is within the first 48 hours; after that time adequate excision is technically much more difficult, and there is also an increased risk of wound infection. Provided the skin graft needed to cover the raw surface can be obtained, all hand burns could be excised regardless of the extent of the total burn surface area, since the operation is performed in a bloodless field.

Treatment before surgery

If immediate surgery is not carried out, the hand is cleaned and a dry compression bandage applied, with 90° flexion in the MP joints and the IP joints extended. The arm is elevated to avoid oedema formation. In the case of very deep dermal and subdermal circumferential burns, escharotomy incisions are made to improve the capillary circulation. These skin incisions should be placed so that tendons are not exposed when the wound edges spread apart. If the fascia must also be split in a concomitant compartment syndrome, it should be incised underneath healthy skin. In the forearm the incision is thus directed towards the ulna in the distal part, both volarly and dorsally. If the carpal tunnel must be released the skin is again incised to the ulnar side, leaving some hypothenar fat in the radial flap, and the most ulnar part of the carpal ligament is divided. In the dorsum of the hand the incisions are placed longitudinally along the first and fourth intermetacarpal spaces. The interossei can then be decompressed by splitting the fascia in all four compartments from these wounds. In the fingers longitudinal incisions are best placed in the mediolateral line on one, or preferably both, sides.

TREATMENT OF DEEP DERMAL BURNS

The operation is performed in a bloodless field under general anaesthesia, or, in the case of localized burns, using regional anaesthesia.

Surgical technique

Tangential excision is carried out with a skin-graft knife. Thin slices are removed down to tissue with normal water content, as observed by the light reflex from the excised surface (Fig. 16.2). One area should be excised down to vital tissue before passing to the next area. The concave surfaces in the interdigital folds and the central parts of the palm are difficult to excise adequately. To facili-

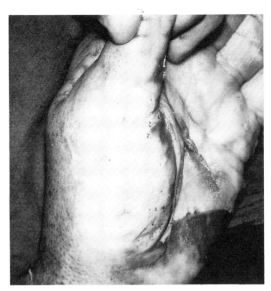

Fig. 16.2 Thumb region after excision, showing light reflex.

tate the excision of the interdigital area or other concave areas, a flexible surgical blade such as Dermagraft can be used. Most cases of dermal burns of the hand involve the dorsum and the thenar and hypothenar regions. Split-skin grafts

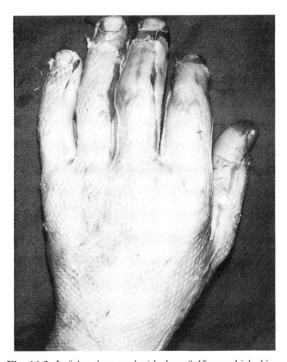

Fig. 16.3 Left hand covered with three 0.45 mm-thick skin grafts with sutures distally on the fingers.

0.45 mm thick are meshed 1.5–1 and then used to cover the primary excised areas of the hands. Meshing is used to prevent blood accumulation between the graft and the excised surface, but the slits in the graft are not expanded. To cover the typical excised area requires three 7 cm × 22 cm grafts. The first graft covers the thumb and the radial part of the hand, the second covers the index and middle fingers and the central part of the hand, and the third covers the ring and little fingers and the ulnar part of the hand. Absorbable sutures are used to suture the grafts distally on to the fingers and in the interdigital folds. Tisseel (fibrin glue) can be used instead of sutures (Fig. 16.3).

Dressing

The graft is covered with Vaseline gauze and cotton compresses moistened with isotonic saline solution. Compression bandage is applied with synthetic wad and a gauze bandage, maintaining 5–10° flexion in the interphalangeal joints, 60–70° flexion in the metacarpophalangeal joints, and 45° wrist extension (Fig. 16.4). After completion of the bandage the tourniquet is released.

Postoperative treatment

The hand is elevated above the level of the heart during the first week. The first dressing change is carried out 3–5 days postoperatively, depending on how long after the injury the excision was done (3 days if not excised during the first 48 hours). Then a similar bandage is reapplied, if possible with maximum flexion in the MP joints. After 1 week physiotherapy is started, using as small a bandage as possible and applying a splint with 90° flexion in the MP joints, straight IP joints and 45° extension in the wrist in between training sessions. In most cases a full range of motion in the affected hand is restored by the end of the second week. When the skin is healed and swelling has subsided, measurements are taken for individually fitted pressure gloves, which are commercially available, to inhibit formation of hypertrophic scars between the grafts. The gloves also protect the skin. The treatment with pressure gloves starts 6–8 weeks after surgery and they are used for a period of at least 6 months (Fig. 16.5).

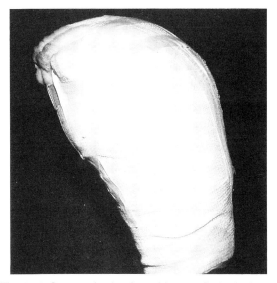

Fig. 16.4 Compression bandage with 5–10° flexion in the interphalangeal joints, 60–70° flexion in the metacarpophalangeal joints, and 45° dorsal flexion in the wrist.

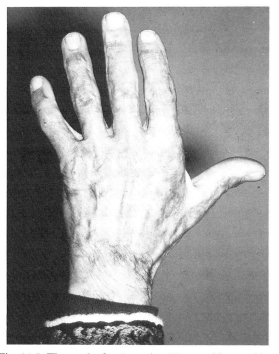

Fig. 16.5 The result after 1 year in a 70-year-old man with a very deep dermal burn.

TREATMENT OF FULL-THICKNESS BURNS

Intact paratenon and/or periosteum

The same technique as above is used and the affected joints are transfixed with Kirschner wires until the skin over the joint is healed.

Without intact paratenon and/or periosteum

In the case of small localized burns, local flaps are taken from an adjacent finger. In extensive burns early or partial amputation should be considered, using volar skin to cover the dorsal side of the finger to preserve finger length. In most cases the burn is much deeper dorsally than volarly. Distant flaps are not used until the excised area is clean.

ELECTRICAL BURNS OF THE HAND

A somewhat wider area is excised because of endothelial capillary damage in the healthy tissue adjacent to the obvious necrosis, which results in a more extensive skin necrosis. The procedure for skin cover is the same as in full-thickness burns. High-tension electrical burns with current flow through the body are always very deep in the regions with small cross-sectional areas, such as the wrist. Angiography is helpful in determining the extent of vessel and muscle damage. Signs of spasm in the vessels always means vessel damage, and the circulation to the hand could cease in a period of 10 days and lead to amputation of the hand. In most cases of high-tension electrical burns, distant flaps are needed to cover the wrist region, and microsurgical repair is not possible because of the damage to large vessels in the forearm.

INCOMPLETE HEALING

Residual raw areas due to defective take of the grafts, or at the borders of the grafts, are usually small and can be left to heal secondarily. If they are larger they must be regrafted.

The surgery is time-consuming, each hand taking 45–90 minutes. However, the need for secondary reconstruction is reduced considerably, especially after deep dermal burns of the hand. Generalized stiffness due to organization of long-standing oedema, as seen when primary healing has not been accomplished, is now seldom met. Thus the primary excision of burns of the hand enhances the healing of the wounds, preserves maximal function and improves the appearance.

REVISION OF BURN SCARS IN THE HAND

After wound healing, scar maturation tends to cause shrinkage of the skin and dermis, giving rise to further loss of the range of motion and sometimes also gross deformity. Secondary scar revision is then necessary to allow the hand to recover potential mobility and function. The principal late skin problems are scars in the interdigital folds and volar scars affecting the extension of the fingers. Where deep structures beneath grafted skin have been damaged, repair of these often requires skin of better quality. Tendon repair and capsulotomy must therefore often be combined with skin Z-plasty, or supple skin must be provided in a preliminary operation before the deep structures are repaired. Revision of burn scars therefore requires additional skin in most cases. Sometimes, however, linear scars may form that can only be released by local Z-plasties.

LOCAL SKIN Z-PLASTIES WITHOUT ADDITIONAL GRAFTING

Such skin Z-plasties are especially useful in the interdigital folds. To widen and deepen the thumb web, a simple Z-plasty may be enough. The best effect is achieved by using the modification of Iselin (1962) (Fig. 16.6) The two right-angle flaps are each divided into two 45° flaps, and these are interdigitated when sutured.

In the other interdigital areas the volar rim of the skin fold is sometimes pulled distally without being scarred. This is usually due to volar lateral shortening of the skin in the finger. Adding length to these areas with Z-plasties will cause the interdigital fold to sink back to its original level. A moderate scar syndactyly may be eliminated by a

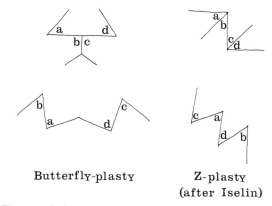

Butterfly-plasty   **Z-plasty**
                           (after Iselin)

Fig. 16.6 Left: butterfly-plasty. Right: Z-plasty, modification of Iselin.

butterfly-plasty (Fig. 16.6) This may be done in a simple interdigital cleft or multiple non-adjacent clefts.

More common is the transverse scar in the dorsal part of the interdigital fold marking the border between grafted skin on the back of the hand and fingers, and intact skin in the thin volar part of the interdigital fold. The local skin plasty may be adequate to release this scar in one interdigital area only if the other interdigital areas have retained their normal slopes.

Volar digital scars may be narrow and the moderate flexion contracture in a finger can then be eliminated by one or two Z-plasties.

SCAR REVISION WITH GRAFTING

As stated above, skin shortage after burns is two-dimensional in most cases, and release of the skin tension very often requires additional skin. When deep structures are involved, well-vascularized flaps may be necessary to cover bone, joints and/or tendons. Capsulotomies and tendon reconstruction may be performed safely at the same time as the skin problem is solved.

Contracture and deformity may be caused by the contracted skin only, in which case free grafts may suffice to restore both function and appearance. On the volar surface full-thickness grafts should be used to hinder the recurrence of scar contracture. This is not a problem on the dorsal aspect of the hand and fingers, where split-skin grafts are satisfactory.

In the palm, incisions to release skin tension are preferably placed along lines that correspond to the flexion creases of the normal palm. The skin grafts should have exactly the same configuration as the defect created by the incision, and the skin margins should be accurately adapted by fine sutures. Some sutures are left with long ends and these are tied over a stent to give some compression to the grafted area. The bandage is left for 8–10 days.

The scarred volar surface of a finger, usually the effect of a contact burn, will cause a flexion deformity of the IP joints. The lateral, often intact, skin is stretched out transversely as the volar scar is bowstringing. In a severe case this lateral skin is incised volarly from the midlateral line at the level of the IP joints, and, if needed, also at the base of the finger. These incisions will meet in the volar midline and triangular flaps are thus formed on each side. After excising or cutting through the subdermal scar tissue the finger can be extended, and the corresponding triangular skin flaps from both sides then overlap the midline. When sutured they form soft skin bridges between diamond-shaped wounds, which are covered with full-thickness skin grafts (Fig. 16.7)

In the interdigital areas soft skin is needed to form the actual folds, and grafted skin is seldom acceptable. A local skin flap from the lateral volar aspect of one finger can be rotated into the dorsal aspect of the interdigital area (MacDougal et al 1976). Its base is cut back to place the volar fold at the normal level. The flap thus has a narrow volar skin pedicle, but with a wider pedicle of subcutaneous tissue, and it turns into the defect in a similar fashion to a rhomboid flap. The length of the flap is calculated so that any transverse tension between the metacarpophalangeal joint projections dorsally is released. The defect formed in the lateral aspect of the finger is grafted.

An extensive scar syndactyly reaching beyond the distal third of the proximal phalanx is best dealt with in the same manner as a congenital syndactyly. A longstanding marked scar contraction of the thumb web will usually require a muscular release. The resulting defect with exposed muscle may still take a full-thickness graft, but in severe cases a distant flap could be introduced.

On the dorsum of the hand burn scars will

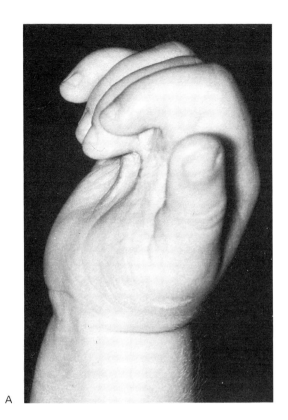

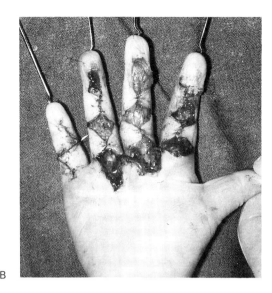

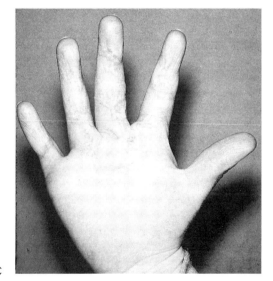

Fig. 16.7 A Severe volar finger contraction after contact burn. **B** Lateral flaps sutured over the midline. Skin defects were covered with full-thickness skin grafts. **C** Full extension after several years.

often hinder flexion of the metacarpophalangeal joints. In severe contracture these will become hyperextended. A capsulotomy is very often necessary as a supplement to skin release, in order to regain flexion. The operation may be planned so that the opened joints are covered with viable skin that has been undermined from a transverse proximal incision. This incision will gape considerably when the metacarpophalangeal joints are flexed, and the split-skin graft should be allowed to heal while the joints are kept in full flexion. Sometimes the contracted dorsal skin is replaced

by extensive hypertrophic scar tissue, and in such a case the total scar should be excised. The wound may extend over the whole dorsum, and is grafted with the MP joints flexed (Fig. 16.8). Transverse skin shortage is most common distally at the MP joint level. If local skin plasties between the MP joints are not sufficient, this area is incised longitudinally. The incision should not cross the volar web distally. The diamond-shaped defect formed is covered with a split-skin graft. Non-elastic scars over the PIP joints are often adherent to underlying extensor tendon, and flexion may

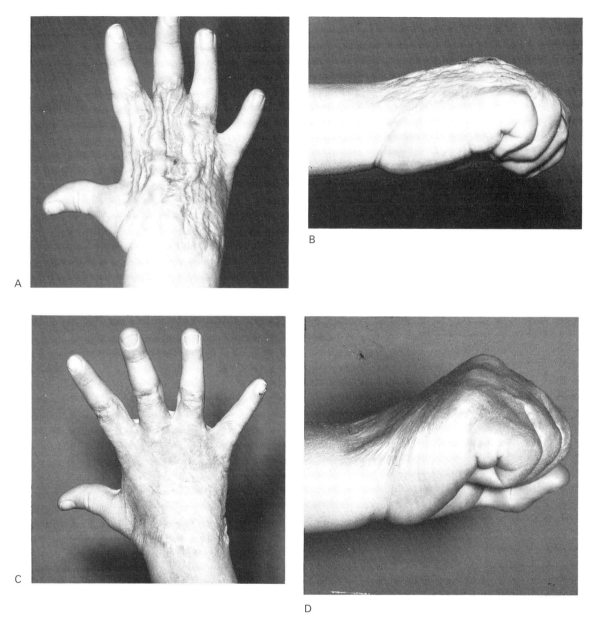

Fig. 16.8 A, B Hypertrophic scar of the dorsum of the hand. **C, D** One year after excision and split-skin grafting.

then be compromised. A skin flap from the lateral side of the middle phalanx, if intact, can supply good coverage over this joint when the scar has been excised. The lateral defect is grafted. Capsulotomy of the PIP joint may also be needed to regain flexion. The nail area is often deformed by burn scarring. The eponychium very often becomes retracted, so that the nail root is exposed. Good

cover can be achieved by lateral flaps based proximally (Barfod 1972) or distally (Ngin & Soin 1986).

FLAP COVER

Deep scarring underneath skin and dermis often demands flap cover. Releasing a flexion contracture of a finger may expose the flexor tendons. A cross-finger flap from the dorsum of an intact adjacent finger is then the best solution. A large defect in the dorsum of the hand due to the excision of hypertrophic scar, when MP joints or extensor tendons are exposed, is best covered with a cross-arm flap using Colson's technique (Colson & Janvier 1966) (see chapter 6). Such a flap can also be used in the case of an extensive thumb adduction contracture.

REFERENCES

Barfod B 1972 Reconstructing the nailfold. Hand 4: 85

Colson P, Janvier H 1966 La dégraissage primaire et total des combeaux d'autoplastie à distance. Annales de Chirurgie Plastique 11: 11

Iselin M 1962 La plastie en Z rectifié. Annales de Chirurgie plastique 7: 295

Jackson D et al 1960 Primary excision and grafting of large burns. Annals of Surgery 152: 167

Jancekovic Z 1970 A new concept in the early excision and immediate grafting of burns. Journal of Trauma 10: 1103

Jancekovic Z 1968 Consistent application of generally adopted surgical principles and the treatment of the burn wound. Present clinical aspects of burns. A symposium. Maribor

MacDougal, Wray, Weeks 1976 Lateral volar fingerflap for the treatment of burn syndactyly. Plastic and Reconstructive Surgery 57: 167

Ngin R G K, Soin K 1986 Postburn nailfold retraction, a reconstructive technique. Journal of Hand Surgery 11B: 385

Index